Aurora Martínez-Romero
José Luis Ortega-Sánchez
Adamas García-Gómez

Occupational implications of lead exposure and health damage.

Aurora Martínez-Romero
José Luis Ortega-Sánchez
Adamas García-Gómez

Occupational implications of lead exposure and health damage.

Pb poisoning. Mechanism of action, toxicokinetics, toxicodynamics, absorption, distribution and accumulation.

ScienciaScripts

Cover image: www.ingimage.com

This book is a translation from the original published under ISBN 978-3-639-48261-4.

Publisher:
Sciencia Scripts
is a trademark of
Dodo Books Indian Ocean Ltd. and OmniScriptum S.R.L publishing group

120 High Road, East Finchley, London, N2 9ED, United Kingdom
Str. Armeneasca 28/1, office 1, Chisinau MD-2012, Republic of Moldova, Europe
Printed at: see last page
ISBN: 978-620-6-28455-0

TABLE OF CONTENTS

FOREWORD

Modern portfolio theory has shown that much of the gain from international diversification comes from the segmentation of financial markets. Stulz (1981a) defines segmentation as the condition where two assets of equal risk, but belonging to two different countries, have different expected returns. In the absence of international barriers, an investor would have to choose the asset with the higher return, thus benefiting from an arbitrage situation.

Markets are said to be fully integrated if assets of the same risk have identical expected returns in all countries. Risk is linked to exposure to a certain common global factor. If a market is segmented from the rest of the world, its covariance with this global factor cannot explain its expected return.

Asset pricing studies can be divided into three groups: segmented markets, integrated markets and partially segmented markets. The first category uses the Capital Asset Pricing Model (CAPM) by Sharpe (1964), Lintner (1965) and Black (1972), and considers financial markets to be segmented.

The second class of asset valuation assumes that financial markets are integrated. These studies are based on the International CAPM (Harvey (1991), the International CAPM with exchange rate risk (Dumas and Solnik (1995) and Dumas (1994)), the model based on world consumption (Wheatley (1988)), international arbitrage valuation theory (Solnik (1983) and Cho et al (1986)), global multi-beta models (Ferson and Harvey (1994), international models with latent variables (Campbell and Hamao (1992), Bekaert and Hodrick (1992) and Harvey, Solnik and Zhou (1994)). The rejection of these models is seen as a rejection of the fundamental model of asset pricing, market inefficiency and integration.

Another part of the literature lies between segmentation and integration. These light segmentation models (Errunza, Losq and Padmanabhan (1992)) do not assume the extreme case of perfect segmentation and perfect integration. The disadvantage of these models is that the degree of segmentation is fixed over time.

Beakaert and Harvey (1995) have proposed a methodology which assumes that the degree of market integration changes over time. Their measure of integration is a time-varying weighting applied to variance and covariance.

In this book, we will study the integration-segmentation of international financial markets. The concept of market integration will be defined, distinguishing financial integration from economic integration. The role of barriers to international investment in market segmentation will be examined. We present various studies designed to test financial integration, highlighting their limitations. A review of the literature will be proposed. Finally, we will attempt to test financial integration for a sample of 15 developed and 7 emerging financial markets over the period (1987-2004) using conditional versions of the CAPM International.

I. FINANCIAL INTEGRATION MEASURES

Financial markets are integrated if two assets whose returns are perfectly correlated in a given currency, but which belong to different countries, have identical expected returns in that currency. Otherwise, markets are said to be segmented, and the investor would take advantage of the difference in returns to invest in the country where the return on risk is highest.

1.1 The concept of market integration

Based on the international arbitrage model, Fontaine (1988) considers financial markets to be economically integrated if, and only if, the same economic factors influence the returns on financial assets in all markets. Financial markets will be financially integrated if, and only if, the risk premiums of the factors expressed in the same currency are identical in all markets. Similarly, for Barari (2004), financial integration implies the absence of a differential between risk premiums on identical assets traded on different financial markets. More generally, two markets are integrated when they evolve in parallel. This means that international diversification is no longer attractive on these markets, due to their high correlations.

According to Aglietta (1991), the integration of financial, monetary or goods and services markets can be defined as the convergence of geographically or sectorally distinct markets towards a single market. Integration generally takes place in stages, due to the difficulty of completely abolishing barriers to integration such as customs barriers, disparities between tax and legal systems, etc. The author has shown that global integration is achieved when international goods and services markets, money markets and financial markets are integrated. Indeed, the integration of goods and services markets requires the absence of customs barriers, the perfect mobility of production factors, as well as the homogeneity of consumer preferences and, consequently, the validity of the law of one price. The integration of financial markets presupposes that there are no barriers to capital flows between countries, and no brokerage fees or other taxes on non-resident investors. This is achieved through interest rate parity. The integration of money markets requires the free operation of currency markets, and in particular the absence of exchange controls.

Dumas (1995) defines a segmented financial market as one in which certain individuals are prohibited from exchanging or holding certain securities. Segmentation generates a form of heterogeneity within the investor population. Indeed, transaction or information costs lead to a differentiation of investors according to the stocks of securities they hold.

La Bruslerie and Mathis (1997) link the problem of capital market integration to asset substitutability and mobility. Two assets are substitutable if they carry identical risks, i.e. if they make the same contribution to the overall risk of a portfolio. In market equilibrium, the expected rates of return on the two assets are identical, and agents are indifferent as to whether they hold one or the other. There is perfect capital mobility, if all agents have identical access to all assets. Obstacles to mobility may be linked to access costs. Rates of return are reduced by a cost, which may be linked either to the existence of transaction costs or different taxes[1] for different investors, or to the existence of information costs[2] .

1.2 Measures based on interest rate parity

International macroeconomics has adopted different methodologies from international finance to measure financial integration. Several researchers, including Frankel and MacArthur (1988) and Frankel (1991), have relied on the interest rate parity condition to measure the financial integration of money markets:

Covered interest rate parity (PTIC): $i_{i,t}^{t+k} = i_{w,t}^{t+k} + (f_t^{t+k} - s_t)$

Unhedged interest rate parity (PTINC) : $i_{i,t}^{t+k} = i_{w,t}^{t+k} + E_t(\Delta s_t^{t+k})$

$$= \left[i_{w,t}^{t+k} + (f_t^{t+k} - s_t)\right] + \left[E_t(\Delta s_t^{t+k}) + (f_t^{t+k} - s_t)\right]$$

Where;

i: nominal interest rate ;

f: forward rate ;

s: spot interest rate.

PTINC is a broader definition of financial integration than PTIC. It takes into account not only the interest-rate risk premium (measured by PTIC), but also the exchange-rate risk premium.

Based on the PTINC relationship, Fratzscher (2002) proposed a measure of financial integration. He derived an uncovered asset return parity relation called Uncovered Asset Return Parity (UAP), to assess the degree of financial integration of the local stock market i into the global stock market w :

$$E_{t-1}\left[r_{i,t}\right] = E_{t-1}\left[r_{w,t}\right] + E_{t-1}\left[\Delta s_{i,t}\right] \quad (1a)$$

[1] Higher costs for non-residents than for residents.

[2] Domestic investors have easier access to information on domestic securities than on foreign securities.

In ex post form, the relationship becomes :

$$r_{i,t} = r_{w,t} + \Delta s_{i,t} \quad (1b)$$

Where;

r : The return on the local currency market portfolio in excess of the risk-free interest rate ;

s_i The spot exchange rate for country i.

The ex-post relationship of asset parity indicates that in a perfectly integrated market, market asset returns r_i are equal to world market asset returns $r_w$and changes in exchange ratesΔs_i.

However, this relationship ignores market and exchange rate risk premiums. In addition, there may be barriers to investment that prevent perfect market integration. This relationship can therefore be rewritten as follows:

$$r_{i,t} = \varphi_{i,t} r_{w,t} + \chi_{i,t} \quad (2)$$

Where;

$\varphi_{i,t}$ the correlation between local yields $r_i$and global yields r_w ;

$\chi_{i,t}$ A vector of country-specific factors.

$\chi_{i,t}$can be broken down into two parts: an anticipated component based on past information $E_{t-1}[r_{i,t}]$ and a non-anticipated component$\varepsilon_{i,t}$i.e. an instantaneous idiosyncratic shock.

$$\chi_{i,t} = \beta_{i,t} E_{t-1}[r_{i,t}] + \varepsilon_{i,t} \quad (3)$$

Similarly, global market returns $r_w$can be expressed in terms of past information $E_{t-1}[r_{w,t}]$and instant innovation $\varepsilon_{w,t}$:

$$\varphi_{i,t} r_{w,t} = \beta_{\text{iw},t} E_{t-1}[r_{w,t}] + \gamma_{\text{iw},t} \varepsilon_{w,t} \quad (4)$$

Substituting the two previous equations into equation (2) gives :

$$r_{i,t} = \beta_{\text{iw},t} E_{t-1}[r_{w,t}] + \gamma_{\text{iw},t} \varepsilon_{w,t} + \beta_{i,t} E_{t-1}[r_{i,t}] + \varepsilon_{i,t} \quad (5)$$

This relationship measures the integration of market i into the global market w. It indicates that local returns$r_{i,t}$are determined on the basis of past information (the expected component of returns) and instantaneous shocks from the local and world markets (the non-expected component).

Indeed, market i is said to be integrated if domestic returns$r_{i,t}$depend on instantaneous world market shocks $\varepsilon_{w,t}$, $\gamma_{\text{iw},t}$therefore measures the degree of integration of market i.

1.3 CAPM-based measurements

Unlike international macroeconomics, the international financial literature has used the CAPM to measure the financial integration of markets (Bekaert and Harvey (1995), Dumas and Solnik (1995), Ferson and Harvey (1991), Hardouvelis et al (1999)...):

$$E_{t-1}(r_{i,t}) = \lambda_w \beta_{\text{iw}} + \lambda_d \beta_{\text{id}} \tag{6}$$

Where;

$r_{i,t}$ The excess return on the portfolio i ;

λ Market risk premium ;

β_{iw} The risk of portfolio i relative to the global market portfolio w ;

β_{id} The risk of portfolio i relative to the domestic market portfolio d.

The null hypothesis of perfect integration requires that $\lambda_d = 0$ i.e. portfolio i is valued only in relation to the global portfolio w. According to this model, expected returns r_i depend solely on non-diversifiable international factors in a perfectly integrated market.

For empirical validation, several econometric methodologies have been adopted. Tests of international linkages between financial markets have mainly been based on VAR models (King and Wadhani (1990) and Eun and Shim (1993)), and have generally highlighted increasing correlations between markets and growing regional interdependence. The most recent research on integration has been conducted within the framework of the GARCH model, in order to take account of the existence of autoregressive effects in high-frequency data. Koutmos and Booth (1995) demonstrated price and volatility increases in the London, Tokyo and New York stock markets. Other studies have focused on time-varying financial integration, modeling time-varying coefficients via instrumental variables. Three instrumental variables are used in the literature. Firstly, it has been shown that the elimination of barriers to capital flows has increased financial integration, not only in developed countries but also in a number of emerging markets (Bekaert and Harvey (1995), Ng (2000)). Secondly, several studies have shown that the degree of real integration, as measured by business cycle correlation, has a significant impact on financial integration (Ferson and Harvey (1991), Jagannathan and Wang (1996)). Thirdly, exchange rate uncertainty has been shown to have a significant impact on financial integration, as exchange rate risk is an important source of risk, which is remunerated in international capital markets (Dumas and Solnik (1995), Hardouvelis et al (1999)).

1.4 The link between economic and financial integration

Several empirical studies have shown that there is a positive long-term relationship between economic activity and stock prices (Fama and French (1988), Schwert (1990), Roll (1992) for the USA and Canova and De Nicole (1995) for European countries).

Based on the present value model, Campbell and Shiller (1988) decomposed the innovations in excess stock returns of different countries into innovations in future excess returns, dividend growth rates, interest rates and exchange rates. By studying the comovements of the different components of excess returns between different countries, it is possible to assess the relative importance of international linkages between economies. In this study, real economic integration is measured by calculating correlations between dividend innovations in different countries, while financial integration is measured by correlations between innovations in expected future stock returns.

Ammer and Mei (1996) developed an approach that measures economic and financial integration by analyzing the covariance of excess returns on national financial markets. The authors measured the financial integration of the two national economies by calculating the correlation between innovations in future expected stock market returns in the two countries. If the financial markets are highly integrated, we should obtain a high correlation between the innovations in future expected returns of the different countries.

Using US and UK data for the period 1957 to 1989, Ammer and Mei (1996) showed that future excess returns are the main source of variation in current stock returns on the New York and London stock exchanges. Similarly, the authors highlighted the existence of high degrees of economic and financial integration between the United States and the United Kingdom. Although future risk premiums explain a large part of the covariance between the stock markets of the different countries, the dividend growth components of the two yields are highly correlated. In addition, the authors show that real and financial linkages became more important after the abolition of the Bretton Woods agreement in the early 1970s. This suggests that increased integration is associated with floating exchange rates.

In the same spirit as Ammer and Mei (1996), Phylaktis and Ravazzolo (2002) examined the role of economic integration in strengthening relations between emerging financial markets. To measure the economic and financial integration of the Basin Pacific countries, the authors decomposed the excess returns of the domestic and foreign markets and their variances. For the domestic market, excess unanticipated returns can be expressed as a linear function of a set of information on future dividend growth rates, real interest rates and excess stock market returns:

$$e_{t+1} - E_t e_{t+1} = (E_{t+1} - E_t)\left\{\sum_{j=0}^{\infty} \rho^j \Delta d_{t+1+j} - \sum_{j=0}^{\infty} \rho^j r_{t+1+j} - \sum_{j=1}^{\infty} \rho^j e_{t+1+j}\right\} \quad (7)$$

Where;

e_{t+1} The return on a share held from the end of period t to the end of period t+1 in excess of the risk-free interest rate.

d_{t+1} The actual dividend paid in period t+1 ;

r_{t+1} The real interest rate from t to t+1 ;

E_t A forecast made at the end of period t, based on a set of data on historical share prices and dividends;

Δ The difference from the previous period ;

ρ A linearization constant.

To simplify equation (7), the authors define the three yield components as follows:

$$\tilde{e} = \tilde{e}_d - \tilde{e}_r - \tilde{e}_e \quad (8)$$

In a similar way, the unanticipated return on a foreign stock in excess of the domestic interest rate ($\tilde{f}$)expressed in dollars, can be decomposed into information on future dividend growth ($\tilde{f}_d$)real interest rates ($\tilde{f}_r$)interest rates, excess stock returns ($\tilde{f}_f$)and changes in the real exchange rate ($\tilde{f}_q$) :

$$(\tilde{f}) = (\tilde{f}_d) - (\tilde{f}_r) - (\tilde{f}_f) - (\tilde{f}_q) \quad (9)$$

Equations (8) and (9) indicate that an increase in future dividends leads to a capital gain, while an increase in expected future returns leads to a capital loss. In equation (9), there is an additional innovation term related to the change in the real exchange rate, which is negatively related to the share's non-expected returns.

These two equations measure the degree of economic and financial integration between two countries. In particular, real economic integration is measured by the correlation between variations in future domestic dividends $\tilde{e}_d$and foreign future dividends$\tilde{f}_d$. Financial integration is measured by the correlation between changes in domestic (future) expected excess returns $\tilde{e}_e$ and foreign returns$\tilde{f}_f$.

Similarly, the variance decomposition of excess unanticipated returns on domestic equities (from equation (8)) can be defined as the sum of six terms:

$$\begin{aligned}\mathrm{Var}(\tilde{e}) = \mathrm{Var}(\tilde{e}_d) - 2\mathrm{Cov}(\tilde{e}_d, \tilde{e}_r) + \mathrm{Var}(\tilde{e}_r) - 2\mathrm{Cov}(\tilde{e}_d, \tilde{e}_e) + \mathrm{Var}(\tilde{e}_e) \\ +2\mathrm{Cov}(\tilde{e}_r, \tilde{e}_e)\end{aligned} \quad (10)$$

Using the decomposition of equation (9), the variance of excess unanticipated foreign equity returns can be defined as the sum of the ten elements:

$$\mathrm{Var}(\tilde{f}) = \mathrm{Var}(\tilde{f}_d) - 2\mathrm{Cov}(\tilde{f}_d, \tilde{f}_r) - 2\mathrm{Cov}(\tilde{f}_d, \tilde{f}_q) - 2\mathrm{Cov}(\tilde{f}_d, \tilde{f}_f) + \mathrm{Var}(\tilde{f}_r) + 2\mathrm{Cov}(\tilde{f}_r, \tilde{f}_q) + 2\mathrm{Cov}(\tilde{f}_r, \tilde{f}_f) + \mathrm{Var}(\tilde{f}_q) + 2\mathrm{Cov}(\tilde{f}_q, \tilde{f}_f) + \mathrm{Var}(\tilde{f}_f) \quad (11)$$

Finally, from equations (8) and (9) it is possible to decompose the covariance of excess returns on domestic and foreign equities as follows:

$$\mathrm{Cov}(\tilde{e}, \tilde{f}) = \mathrm{Cov}(\tilde{e}_d, \tilde{f}_d) - \mathrm{Cov}(\tilde{e}_d, \tilde{f}_r) - \mathrm{Cov}(\tilde{e}_d, \tilde{f}_q) - \mathrm{Cov}(\tilde{e}_d, \tilde{f}_f) - \mathrm{Cov}(\tilde{e}_r, \tilde{f}_d) + \mathrm{Cov}(\tilde{e}_r, \tilde{f}_r) + \mathrm{Cov}(\tilde{e}_r, \tilde{f}_q) + \mathrm{Cov}(\tilde{e}_r, \tilde{f}_f) - \mathrm{Cov}(\tilde{e}_e, \tilde{f}_d) + \mathrm{Cov}(\tilde{e}_e, \tilde{f}_r) + \mathrm{Cov}(\tilde{e}_e, \tilde{f}_q) + \mathrm{Cov}(\tilde{e}_e, \tilde{f}_f) \quad (12)$$

The estimation results for the United States (domestic country) and Japan, Hong Kong, Indonesia, Korea, Malaysia, Philippines, Singapore, Taiwan and Thailand (foreign countries) during the two periods 1980.01-1989.12 and 1990.01-1998.12 are as follows:

Firstly, the variation in dividends is the largest component of the variance in the returns of the countries examined. The contribution of the risk premium is much smaller. Similarly, the correlation between future dividend growth for each country pair is the largest source of covariance in domestic and foreign equity returns, demonstrating the importance of economic integration in the region. What's more, this integration seems to have strengthened during the 1990s for the countries of the Pacific Basin.

Secondly, the high and statistically significant covariance between domestic excess returns and foreign future dividends shows the interaction between economic and financial integration.

Thirdly, an examination of the correlation matrix of returns shows that during the 1990s, all the countries in the Pacific Basin were financially and economically integrated. There was regional economic and financial integration, even before the Asian crisis. These results confirm the idea that economic integration and trade interdependence can play a major role in the contagion effect of the Asian crisis. What's more, some countries have close ties with the United States, while others have close ties with Japan. Thailand, for example, is highly integrated with the USA, while Korea and Taiwan have strong ties with Japan.

Kim, Moshirian and Wu (2006) examined the dynamic relationship between the daily stock and bond returns of Eurozone countries (Germany, France, Spain and Italy) and non-Eurozone countries (USA, Japan and UK) over the period 2/3/1994 to 9/19/2003, in order to study the progress of financial integration between the markets. The authors empirically investigated the influence of the European Monetary Union on the time-varying dynamics of bond and stock market integration/segmentation, using a two-stage procedure: First, they examined trends in conditional time-varying correlations between bond and stock market returns in European countries, the USA and Japan. Secondly, they studied the causality and determinants of this interdependent relationship, in particular the role of the European Monetary Union. By modeling the process by which bond and stock market returns are generated with an E-GARCH model[3] , taking into account positive and negative shocks to returns, the results of empirical tests show that real economic integration and the reduction of exchange rate risk have a favorable effect on financial integration.

[3] Exponential Generalized Autoregressive Conditional Heteroscedasticity.

II. Barriers to international investment and the segmentation of financial markets

The existence of barriers to international investment has an impact on the share of foreign assets in investors' portfolios, which could lead to the segmentation of capital markets.

The financial literature has shown that, in the presence of constraints on international investment, the assets available to foreign investors command higher prices than those available to domestic investors. In this section, we propose the models of Eun and Janakiramanan (1986), Hietala (1989), Domowitz, Glen and Madhavan (1997), Foerester and Karolyi (1999), Chen, Lee and Rui (2001) and Stulz and Wasserfallen (1985).

2.1 Eun and Janakiramanan's model (1986)

Eun and Janakiramanan (1986) proposed a model that characterizes market segmentation as a restriction imposed by the foreign government on domestic investors. This restriction is characterized by the fixing of a well-defined proportion to hold assets of foreign companies, in order to keep their control in the hands of local investors. Eun and Janakiramanan's (1986) model assumes the existence of two countries in the world economy, which is a simplifying assumption, but it does not fundamentally alter the reasoning. The authors also show that, in the absence of any form of restriction, domestic asset prices are the same for all investors in the global economy.

In fact, the expected return on a domestic asset is given by the following relationship :

$$R = r + \lambda^{-1} M \mathrm{cov}(R_i, R_m) \quad (13)$$

Where;

r: risk-free interest rate ;

λ Risk aversion among domestic and foreign investors;

M: market capitalization of the domestic market.

The previous relationship shows that assets have the same return for all investors. The presence of restrictions on the number of assets held by investors is denoted byθ. The return on foreign securities is not similar for the two types of investor. Thus, for a domestic investor, the return on a restricted asset is given by :

$$R = r + \lambda^{-1} M \mathrm{cov}(R_i, R_m) + (\lambda^{-1} - (\lambda^C)^{-1}\theta)\left[\mathrm{cov}(R_{i,}R_I) - \mathrm{cov}(R_i, R_e)\right] \quad (14)$$

Where;

λ^c Risk aversion among forced foreign investors ;

λ^{nc} Risk aversion of unconstrained domestic investors;

R_iThe return on constrained assets;

R_e : the return on unconstrained assets ;

R_I The market portfolio of constrained assets;

r: return on risk-free assets.

This return is not the same for the foreign investor, as shown by the following relationship:

$$R = r + \lambda^{-1} M \text{cov}(R_i, R_m) + ((\lambda^{nc})^{-1}(1-\theta) - \lambda^{-1})\left[\text{cov}(R_{i,}R_I) - \text{cov}(R_i, R_e)\right] \quad (15)$$

From relations (3.14) and (3.15), we can see that investors do not have the same return.

Eun and Janakiramanan (1986) show that the asset price for both categories of investors is equal to the equilibrium price (P*), plus a risk premium for domestic investors. The price of the same asset is equal to the equilibrium price minus a discount for foreign investors, which translates into :

$$P_I^c = P_I^* + \varphi \quad (16)$$

Where;

φ the premium for domestic investors.

$$P_I^{nc} = P_I^* - v \quad (17)$$

Where;

v deportation for foreign investors.

This shows that segmentation provides a different return and price for the same asset for domestic investors.

2.2 Hietala's model (1989)

Hietala (1989) proposes a model of international valuation in the presence of three types of assets on the market. In this model, the world economy is made up of two countries. On the domestic market, there is a single type of asset (called A) specific to local investors. The foreign market is characterized by two kinds of assets called B, which can be held by all investors, particularly domestic investors, and assets C which are available only to investors from foreign countries (constrained assets).

In this model, Hietala (1989) shows that assets A and B, which constitute the domestic investor's set of investment opportunities $(A \cup B = G)$are evaluated by the following relationship :

$$R_g \leq r + \beta_g(R_G - r) \qquad \forall g \in G \tag{18}$$

Where;

R_G expected equilibrium return on the domestic market portfolio ;

$\beta_g = \frac{\text{cov}(R_g,R_G)}{\text{var}R_G}$ Asset beta g ;

r: return on risk-free assets.

In fact, the previous relationship can be broken down into two valuation relationships. The first allows us to value the assets held at equilibrium, called G*, by the domestic investor:

$$R_{g*=r+\beta_{g*(R_G-r)} \quad \forall g*G*} \tag{19}$$

Where;

R_{g*} expected return on asset g* at equilibrium ;

R_G : the expected return on the market portfolio of the domestic country ;

$\beta_g = \text{cov}(R_{g*\frac{,R_{G*})}{\text{var}R_{G*}}}$ beta of asset g*.

Assets not held by the domestic investor are valued at equilibrium using the following relationship:

$$R_g \leq r + \beta_g(R_G - r) \qquad \forall g \in G - G* \tag{20}$$

Similarly, assets held H* at equilibrium by foreign investors are valued by the following relationship :

$$R_{h*=r+\beta_{h*(R_H-r)} \quad \forall h*H*} \tag{21}$$

Where;

R_{h*} expected equilibrium return on asset h ;

R_H : the expected return on the foreign country's market portfolio ;

$\beta_{h*} = \frac{\text{cov}(R_{h*,},R_{H*})}{\text{var}R_{H*}}$ asset beta h* ;

$(B \cup C = H)$ the pool of assets available to foreign investors.

Foreign assets not held by foreign investors are valued using the following relationship:

$$R_h \leq r + \beta_h(R_G - r) \qquad \forall h \in H - H^* \tag{22}$$

Using Hietala's (1989) model, we can see that assets A, B and C do not generate the same risk premium. In fact, this premium varies from asset to asset. Type B assets provide the same risk premium for both domestic and foreign investors. The difference between the risk premium associated with assets A and C is one explanation for investors' tendency to choose international portfolios. In conclusion, barriers to international investment help explain investor behavior.

2.3 The Stulz and Wasserfallen (1995) model and the Domowitz, Glen and Madhavan (1997) model

Stulz and Wasserfallen (1995) have shown that stocks that differ only in their accessibility to foreign investors trade at significantly different prices, and that the most accessible stocks sell at higher prices.

The authors show that the constraints imposed on investors play a role in portfolio choice. Indeed, the demand for domestic assets by domestic and foreign investors is not the same. This function depends on the costs incurred by the investor to participate in the foreign market. Their model presents two important results:

- ✓ it is optimal for the company to sell shares to foreign investors at a higher price, if the price elasticity of demand of these investors is lower than that of domestic investors.
- ✓ price discrimination is a necessary and sufficient condition for maximizing firm value.

The model of Stulz and Wasserfallen (1995) shows that demand for assets by domestic investors is more price-elastic than demand from foreign investors, and that the price of assets available to foreign investors is higher than those available to domestic investors. This result is confirmed empirically by a study of the Swiss market.

In the same spirit of analysis, Domowitz, Glen and Madhavan (1997) examined the impact of foreign investment constraints on share prices in the Mexican stock market. The financial literature has shown the existence of premiums on the prices of unconstrained stocks (accessible to both domestic and foreign investors) compared with constrained stocks (accessible only to domestic investors). These results can be grouped into two model categories: the differential valuation model and the liquidity model.

Differential valuation models assume that price differences arise from higher valuations by foreign investors (compared to domestic investors) of the firm's expected cash flows, due to differences in risk attitudes, tax rates, etc. These models include the case where the demand functions of domestic and foreign investors are different because information costs vary between countries. These models include the case where the demand functions of domestic and foreign investors are different, as information costs vary between countries.

Let's assume that P_A represents the price of A shares available only to Mexican investors and S_A represents the number of A shares. B shares are available to all investors. Since domestic investors can buy either A or B shares, these investors will hold A shares, whereas foreign investors can only hold B shares, even if they are traded at a premium to B shares. To explain the premium on share prices, the authors assume that the firm pays a dividend on both constrained and unconstrained shares. θ on both constrained and unconstrained shares. Domestic and foreign investors maximize mean-variance expected utility functions. Demand functions are assumed to be linear and take the following form for domestic and foreign investors respectively:

$$d_A = \alpha(v_d - p_A)$$

$$d_B = \beta(v_f - p_B)$$

In these demand functions, α and β are positive constants and v_d and $v_f$are evaluations of the company's expected dividends. Formally, $v_d = E_d[\theta] - 2A_d\sigma_d$ where$A_d$is the coefficient of absolute risk aversion for domestic investors and σ_d is the covariance between the stochastic dividend and domestic investors' asset income, likewise, $v_f = E_f[\theta] - 2A_f\sigma_f$. Using the properties of the expected utility function, we can write that $\alpha = N_d/2\,A_d\sigma^2_{d,\theta}$ and $\beta = N_f/2\,A_f\sigma^2_{f,\theta}$ with $N_d(N_f)$is the number of domestic (foreign) investors and $\sigma^2_{d,\theta}\left(\sigma^2_{f,\theta}\right)$ is the conditional variance of asset income for domestic (foreign) investors. Thus, the coefficients of demand α and β decrease with risk aversion and perceptions of asset variance, and increase with the number of investors.

In this model, the ratio of unconstrained to constrained stock prices is expressed as follows:

$$\frac{p_B}{p_A} = \left(\frac{v_f - \beta^{-1}S_B}{v_d - \alpha^{-1}S_A}\right) \tag{23}$$

This equation indicates that an increase in the number of foreign investors[4] will necessarily lead to an increase in the premium. Similarly, an increase in the risk aversion of foreign investors or in the perceived volatility of the asset will lead to a decrease in β and reduce the premium.

With regard to the liquidity model, the price premiums on unconstrained B shares reflect the low transaction costs and high liquidity of these shares compared with A shares.

Let's assume that $2\varphi_A$ represents the bid-ask-spread percentage in A shares and $2\varphi_B$in B shares. Therefore, the buyer of the share pays the ask price of $p(1+\varphi)$at the end of the period,

[4] This means an increase inβ.

and receives the bid price of $v(1-\varphi)$. For an investor to be indifferent between the two markets, the returns net of the costs of buying A or B shares must be identical. This implies that :

$$\left(\frac{v(1-\varphi_B)}{p_B(1+\varphi_B)}\right)=\left(\frac{v(1-\varphi_A)}{p_A(1+\varphi_A)}\right) \tag{24}$$

Rearranging this equation gives :

$$\frac{p_B}{p_A}=\left(\frac{1+\varphi_A}{1+\varphi_B}\right)\left(\frac{1-\varphi_B)}{1-\varphi_A)}\right) \tag{25}$$

This equation indicates that the equity price premium is an increasing function of the relative transaction costs in markets A and B.

Empirical analysis of the Mexican market, based on monthly observations over the period 1990-1993, shows the existence of a statistically and economically significant premium for unconstrained stocks over constrained stocks, suggesting that barriers to foreign investment lead to market segmentation.

To analyze temporal and cross-sectional variations in the equity price premium, and to distinguish between the liquidity hypothesis and the price discrimination hypothesis, the authors developed a panel data model. The empirical results support the hypothesis of Stulz and Wasserfallen (1995), underlining the relative scarcity of unconstrained stocks. They also indicate that price premiums on unconstrained stocks are not the result of differential market liquidity.

2.4 The study by Chen, Lee and Rui (2001)

Chen, Lee and Rui (2001) examined the effect of foreign ownership constraints on share prices in China. Since the establishment of the Shanghai Stock Exchange in 1990 and the Shenzhen Stock Exchange in 1991, China's financial markets have expanded rapidly. Many companies issue two types of shares. Type A shares are traded between domestic investors, while type B shares can be held by foreign investors. Unlike in other countries, B shares are sold at a lower price than A shares. Indeed, based on a sample of 68 companies with both A and B shares, the authors showed that A-share prices exceeded B-share prices by 66.2% on the Shanghai Stock Exchange and 52.4% on the Shenzhen Stock Exchange over the period 1992-1997. Similarly, they show that the A-share market is expanding relative to the B-share market. It is also more liquid and more active.

To explain the price differential between shares A and B, Chen, Lee and Rui (2001) examine four hypotheses: the information asymmetry hypothesis, the differential demand hypothesis, the liquidity hypothesis and the risk differential hypothesis.

Concerning information asymmetry, Chakravarty, Sarkar and Wu (1998) have shown that the difference between A and B share prices is linked to the difficulties encountered by foreign investors in acquiring and evaluating information on local Chinese companies. To evaluate this hypothesis, Chen, Lee and Rui (2001) carried out causality tests of returns and return volatilities between A and B shares. If the asymmetric information hypothesis holds, A-share returns should drive B-share returns and vice versa. Furthermore, several studies (Anderson (1996)) suggest that information flows between the two share classes can be studied by examining the volatility of returns. If this hypothesis holds, then the premium on B shares falls if the information asymmetry is reduced.

The differential demand hypothesis is based on the model by Stulz and Wasserfallen (1995), and assumes that demand functions for domestic equities differ between domestic and foreign investors. In this model, the difference between share prices is smaller if foreign demand increases. This suggests that price discrimination is a negative function of foreign investors' demand for stocks A and B.

The liquidity hypothesis states that the price differential is due to the low liquidity of B shares and their high transaction costs. Amihud and Mendelson (1986) suggest that relatively illiquid stocks have a higher expected return and a lower price to compensate for higher transaction costs. According to the liquidity hypothesis, the price differential is an inverse function of thc liquidity of B shares relative to A shares.

The risk differential hypothesis indicates that Chinese and foreign investors have different risk aversions. The international asset pricing models of Eun and Janakiramanan (1986) show that price differences can be explained by investors' risk attitudes, the difference between domestic and foreign risk-free rates, the liquidity and correlation of different stocks, and changes in regulation.

In particular, Chinese markets are highly speculative, and investors are very risk-tolerant and want to make money quickly. The speculative behavior of Chinese investors can boost A-share prices. Consequently, the difference in investors' risk aversion could explain the fall in B share prices.

Chen, Lee and Rui (2001) attempted to analyze these hypotheses empirically using a panel data model (same methodology as Domowitz, Glen and Madhavan (1997)). All hypotheses were rejected, with the exception of liquidity. The analysis indicates that the price differential is negatively correlated with the ratio of B-share trading volume to total trading volume. Therefore, illiquid B shares have a lower price to compensate for the high level of transaction costs.

III. Valuation of assets with time-varying degrees of integration

International asset pricing models suggest that portfolio flow barriers affect the degree and temporal variation of global financial market integration.

3.1 The Bekaert and Harvey model (1995)

Bekaert and Harvey (1995) have proposed a model that combines the hypothesis of perfect integration with that of perfect segmentation, and determines the probability (time-varying) that the market structure will conform to one of the two regimes.

Using a sample of 12 emerging markets over the period from December 1975 to December 1992, the model's estimation results indicate that the degree of integration varies over time for most countries.

Bekaert and Harvey (1995) have shown that the Greek market is integrated into world capital markets. Its integration parameter was 0.86 during the 1990s. This result is consistent with Greece's investment environment. Indeed, outside certain industries, such as banking, insurance and fishing, there are no constraints on foreign investment. Similarly, the Korean market has become integrated into the world market in recent years. During the 1990s, the integration parameter rose to 0.99. The existence of country funds has enabled foreigners to access the Korean market. For Malaysia, the results indicate that the market is integrated, with a parameter of 0.79 during the 1990s. Foreigners play an important role in the Malaysian market. At the end of 1992, foreign participation stood at 27%.

The results for Mexico appear to be surprising. The model estimates suggest that the market is segmented, with the exception of the 1982-1985 period and the late 1980s, with a trend towards integration from 1991 onwards with the liberalization of the stock market.

Model estimates for Thailand show an increase in the probability of integration from 1986 onwards. In 1992, foreign ownership was estimated at 60% of shares. This market has a large market capitalization, is highly liquid and had the second-highest turnover ratio among emerging markets in 1992. In Zimbabwe, the market is not perfectly integrated, with an average integration rate of 57% in the 90s, compared with zero in the mid-80s, due to the existence of exchange controls.

The Chilean market exhibits a certain degree of segmentation. Foreign investors must pay a 35% tax on dividends and capital gains. In addition, there are exchange controls, and the official rate diverges from the market rate. Most foreign investment flows must use the official rate.

The results for Colombia suggest that the market is segmented, which is consistent with the country's investment environment. Low market liquidity combined with political risk (drug cartels), explains the segmentation of the Colombian market.

The Indian market is not fully integrated into global capital markets. Foreign investors need authorization from the Indian central bank to acquire shares. Other factors, such as political and religious conflicts and tensions with Pakistan, militate against foreign investor participation in the Indian market.

The Jordanian market is not perfectly integrated into world capital markets. In 1992, 85% of shares were owned by Jordanians and 15% by investors from other Arab countries. There are no ADRs or country funds. Direct purchase of shares is the only way to access the Jordanian market.

Finally, the Nigerian study shows that the market is highly segmented. Low market liquidity and the non-existence of Nigerian ADRs and Country Funds explain the results obtained.

3.2 The Carrieri, Errunza and Hogan (2007) model

The results of Bekaert and Harvey (1995) are confirmed by a more recent study by Carrieri, Errunza and Hogan (2007). The latter assessed the time varying integration of emerging financial markets by estimating the Errunza and Losq (1985) model, which assumes that market structure lies between perfect integration and perfect segmentation.

More specifically, Carrieri, Errunza and Hogan (2007) constructed an integration index based on the Errunza and Losq (1985) model. In this model, the integration/segmentation hypothesis was tested on the basis of this relationship:

$$E(R_i) = R_f + \text{AMCov}(R_i, R_w) + (A_I - A)M_I\text{Cov}(R_i, R_I|\underline{R_e}) \qquad (26a)$$

This relationship indicates that the expected return on i[ème] assets has a global risk premium and a super-risk premium which is proportional to the risk of the conditional market. Securities that are bought without constraints by any investor will be valued as if the markets were fully integrated, i.e. they will not require any super-risk premium.

By aggregating this relationship with all ineligible (constrained) securities, we obtain the following expression:

$$E(R_I - R_f) = \text{AMCov}(R_I, R_w) + (A_u - A)M_I\text{Var}(R_I|\underline{R_e}) \qquad (26b)$$

Based on conditional market risk, which is interpreted as a measure of substitutability between an ineligible security and the entire eligible segment of the global market, Carrieri, Errunza and Hogan (2007) have developed a measure of substitution for all ineligible securities, called the Integration Index :

$$\text{Indice d'Intégration} = \text{I I} = 1 - \frac{\text{Var}(R_I|\underline{R_e})}{\text{Var}(R_I)} \tag{27}$$

By definition, this index varies between 0 and 1. In the extreme case of perfect integration, the integration index is equal to 1, i.e. $\text{Var}(R_I|\underline{R_e}) = 0$There is an eligible security (or combination of securities) that is perfectly correlated with the market portfolio of ineligible securities. In this case, equation (26b) states that there is no super-risk premium and that the two market segments are effectively integrated. The market lines for securities in all countries are identical, and the only measure of risk is the beta coefficient defined in relation to the world market portfolio. In particular, the required return on the market portfolio of ineligible securities is determined exclusively by the global risk aversion coefficient and the systematic risk of ineligible securities.

$$E(R_I) = R_f + \text{AMCov}(R_I, R_w) \tag{28}$$

In the case of perfect segmentation, the integration index is zero, i.e.$\text{Var}(R_I|\underline{R_e}) = \text{Var}(R_I)$. The conditional and unconditional variances are equal, and the correlation between the return on the market portfolio of ineligible securities and the return on any eligible security or portfolio is zero, $\text{Cov}(R_I, \underline{R_e}) = 0$.

$$E(R_I) = R_f + A_u M_I \text{Var}(R_I) \tag{29}$$

In this case, the expected return on the portfolio of ineligible securities is determined by the variance of returns, not by the covariance with the return on the global market portfolio. In other words, the presence of constrained investors and eligible securities in the market will have no effect on the overall market value of ineligible securities.

Carrieri, Errunza and Hogan (2007) have constructed diversification portfolios (DP), measuring the ability of internationally traded assets (ADRs and Country Funds) to substitute foreign assets. The DP is defined as the portfolio of eligible securities that is most highly correlated with the market portfolio of ineligible securities:

$$\text{Var}(R_I|\underline{R_e}) = \text{Var}(R_I)(1 - \rho_{I,e}^2) \tag{30}$$

Where;

$\rho_{I,e}$ the correlation coefficient between R_I and the diversification portfolio.

Note that if $\rho_{I,e}$ 1the diversification (domestic) portfolio is perfectly correlated with the foreign market portfolio.

To estimate Errunza and Losq's (1985) model, Carrieri, Errunza and Hogan (2007) used GARCH methodology to empirically determine the time variation of market integration. Based on the stock market indices of 8 emerging markets (Argentina, Brazil, Chile, India, Korea, Mexico, Taiwan and Thailand) over the period 1976-2000, the results suggest that, while local risk is the only relevant factor in explaining the time variation of emerging market returns, global risk is conditionally rewarded in Mexico, Taiwan and Brazil, and is of marginal significance in India and Argentina. Furthermore, the results show significant differences in the degree of integration in the various countries. Mexico is the most integrated market in the sample, while Argentina is the most segmented. The study also indicates that, for all the countries examined, the degree of integration increased significantly during the 90s, due to the reduction of barriers to portfolio flows, the liberalization of capital markets and the introduction of ADRs and country funds on American stock exchanges.

IV. Market segmentation and the cost of capital in international capital markets

Financial market reforms and liberalization in developed economies in the 1970s, and in emerging economies in the late 1980s, removed a number of barriers to international investment. Deregulation and the development of local stock markets have created favorable conditions for attracting foreign portfolio investment. Empirical studies have shown that capital market liberalization reduces the cost of capital. Indeed, this cost is the discount rate used to discount the expected cash flows from a firm's project, and is none other than the rate of return demanded by shareholders, as determined by the CAPM. If a financial market is segmented from the international market, the required rate of return is equal to the risk-free rate plus a risk premium (a firm's beta multiplied by the local market risk premium). However, as markets open up, investors will benefit from liberalization through diversification, as some domestic and foreign risks offset each other (Stulz (1999)). Consequently, we might expect a reduction in the rate of return demanded of domestic investors, and hence a lower cost of capital as a result of reduced risk.

Henry (1998) analyzed the liberalization of 12 emerging markets and showed that stock market returns increased by 39% with liberalization. Errunza, Senbet and Hogan (1998) showed theoretically that the introduction of Country Funds reduces the cost of capital of underlying assets. This is because Country Funds allow investors to substitute foreign yields with domestically traded securities.

Bekaert and Harvey (2000) examined the impact of financial liberalization on the process of generating stock market returns in 20 emerging markets. Given the complexity of the liberalization process, the authors defined capital market liberalization using three alternative measures: formal regulatory liberalization, the date of issue of the first ADR or Country Fund, and the date of structural change in capital flows (increase in flows). Due to the high volatility of returns and the uncertainty associated with capital market liberalization dates, the authors used dividend yields instead of average returns to measure changes in the cost of capital. Empirical analysis indicates that dividend yields fall after liberalization, but the effect is on average less than 1%.

In addition, correlations and betas with the global market have risen steadily since the start of liberalization, with the exception of three countries (out of a sample of 20 emerging countries) which have seen a slight decline. This increase was very significant at the end of the 90s, reflecting greater market integration and higher global volatility.

Errunza and Miller (2000) have studied the impact of foreign ownership on the cost of capital through the introduction of ADRs. To assess the change in the cost of capital, it is important to know the nature of the market. If the domestic market I is completely segmented from the global market, the underlying firm must be valued as follows:

$$E(R_i) = R_f + A_I M_I \mathrm{Cov}(R_i, R_I) \tag{31}$$

Where;

$E(R_i)$ the expected return on asset i in the domestic market I ;

R_f risk-free interest rate ;

A_I the risk aversion coefficient of market investors I ;

$M_I(R_I)$ value (return) of market portfolio I.

Thus, the expected return depends on the national covariance risk.

With the introduction of ADR on the world market, the company will be valued with full integration. The valuation relationship of CAPM International in the absence of currency risk will be :

$$E(R_i) = R_f + \mathrm{AMCov}(R_i, R_w) \tag{32}$$

Where;

A global risk aversion coefficient ;

$M(R_w)$ value (return) of the global market portfolio.

Thus, expected returns depend on international covariance risk. In general, we should expect the price of global risk to be lower than the price of local risk, the global market portfolio to be less volatile than the local market portfolio, and securities to be more correlated within the same market than between international financial markets. Therefore, the expected return (or cost of capital) of a stock in the segmented market should fall following the introduction of an ADR valued in an integrated market.

However, financial markets are neither fully segmented nor fully integrated, and it is with this in mind that Errunza and Miller (2000) have used a model of light segmentation where I market investors can trade all assets and other investors can only trade domestic assets. In this case, the valuation relationship will be :

$$E(R_i) = R_f + \mathrm{AMCov}(R_i, R_w) + (A_I - A) M_I \mathrm{Cov}(R_i, R_I | \underline{R_e}) \tag{33}$$

Where;

$\underline{R_e}$ the vector of returns on all securities that can be traded by all investors, regardless of their nationality.

The expected return on i[ème] shares is made up of a global risk premium and a super-risk premium, which is proportional to the conditional market risk, $\mathrm{Cov}(R_i, R_I|\underline{R_e})$.

In the case of two countries, we can consider the I market as a developed or emerging market, and the other country as the US market. The vector $\underline{R_e}$will therefore be made up of all the securities traded on the US market, and the conditional market risk will depend on the ability of US investors to obtain the benefits of international diversification without investing abroad. Indeed, the existence of substitute assets on the domestic market reduces the diversification potential of the firm introducing the ADR. If US investors can perfectly duplicate the return on 1 foreign assets via domestic diversification[5] , then the super-risk premium will disappear. In the other extreme case, if correlation is zero, all else being equal, stock i would require a higher expected return to reach diversification potential.

In line with the empirical literature on tests of international CAPM predictions and the segmentation hypothesis, the authors used a measure based on realized returns to study changes in the long-term cost of capital, following the announcement of ADR. Similarly, following the methodology of Bekaert and Harvey (2000), Errunza and Miller (2000) used changes in dividend yields[6] during liberalization for a sample of 126 companies belonging to 32 developed and emerging countries. The results are as follows:

Firstly, realized returns fall by 42.2% after liberalization, indicating a reduction in the cost of capital. Furthermore, the results based on dividend yields are similar and consistent with those based on realized returns. These results at firm level[7] are in line with the studies carried out at market level.

Secondly, realized returns were high prior to the announcement of liberalization, indicating that markets were segmented with a higher risk premium and therefore a fairly high cost of capital.

Thirdly, the study suggests that just after liberalization, asset valuations increase considerably. This upward adjustment in asset values is due to the fall in the cost of capital. This economically and statistically significant decline depends on the diversification potential of the foreign firm, as predicted by international CAPMs.

[5] That is, the correlation between the returns of the 1 asset and the domestic diversification portfolio is close to unity.
[6] The dividend yield is used as a proxy for the change in the cost of capital.
[7] This study examines the impact of liberalization and foreign participation on the cost of capital via the introduction of ADR at the firm level, whereas studies such as Henry (1998) and Bekaert and Harvey (2000a) consider liberalization dates at the market level.

Finally, the cost of capital for firms in developed markets is higher than for firms in emerging markets. Overall, the results validate the hypothesis that market liberalization offers significant economic benefits in terms of the cost of capital.

Jong and De Roon (2005) also examined the effects of liberalization on the cost of capital in emerging markets. They assumed that there are two categories of assets: eligible assets, which can be held by all investors, and ineligible assets, which are held only by domestic investors.

For an investor in an emerging market j, the first-order conditions are expressed as follows:

$$\lambda^j \begin{bmatrix} \mu_I \\ \mu_X \end{bmatrix} = \begin{bmatrix} \sum \mathrm{II} & \sum \mathrm{IX} \\ \sum \mathrm{XI} & \sum \mathrm{XX} \end{bmatrix} \begin{bmatrix} \omega_I^j \\ \omega_X^j \end{bmatrix}$$

Where;

λ^j The inverse of the representative investor's risk aversion;

μ_I expected returns on eligible (unconstrained) assets ;

μ_X : expected returns on ineligible assets (restricted to investors)

foreigners) ;

$\sum$ II variance of returns on eligible assets ;

$\sum$ IX the covariance between returns on eligible and ineligible assets ;

$\sum$ XX variance of returns on ineligible assets.

Aggregated for all agents (countries), the risk premium of eligible assets is given by the following equation :

$$E_t\left[r_{i,t+1}^I\right] = \gamma^m \mathrm{Cov}_t\left[r_{i,t+1}^I, r_{t+1}^w\right]\left(1 - \sum q_{j,t}^m\right) + \gamma^m \sum_{j=1}^K \mathrm{Cov}_t\left[r_{i,t+1}^I, r_{j,t+1}^X\right] q_{j,t}^m \quad (34)$$

Where;

γ^m Global risk aversion;

r_{t+1}^w : the return on the global market portfolio of eligible assets ;

$q_{j,t}^m$ the segmentation variable for country j; it is defined by :

$$q_{j,t}^m = \frac{Y_t^j w_X^j}{\sum_{k=1}^K Y_t^k} = \frac{Q_t^j}{Y_t^M}$$

This segmentation variable represents the market value of ineligible assets (Q_t^j)in relation to that of all assets (Y_t^M)worldwide.

The first term in equation (34) is none other than the standard International CAPM, and the second term represents the risk premium if the asset provides a hedge against the risk of ineligible asset returns. This model can be written as a function of beta:

$$E_t\left[r_{i,t+1}^I\right] = \beta_i E_t\left[r_{t+1}^w\right] + \sum_{j=1}^K \theta_{\text{ij}}\, q_{j,t}^m \tag{35a}$$

Or ;

$$\beta_i = \frac{\text{Cov}\left[r_{i,t+1}^I, r_{t+1}^w\right]}{\text{Var}\left[r_{t+1}^w\right]} \tag{35b}$$

$$\theta_{\text{ij}} = \gamma^m \text{Cov}\left[r_{i,t+1}^I, r_{j,t+1}^w\right] - \beta_i \text{Cov}\left[r_{t+1}^w, r_{j,t+1}^X\right] \tag{35c}$$

This model is a generalization of CAPM International, where the additional terms represent the shares of non-traded assets in all countries relative to total assets worldwide.

For ineligible assets, we can obtain a similar valuation relationship:

$$E_t\left[r_{i,t+1}^X\right] = \beta_j E_t\left[r_{t+1}^I\right] + \phi_j q_t^j \tag{36a}$$

Where;

$$\beta_j = \frac{\text{Cov}\left[r_{i,t+1}^X, r_{t+1}^I\right]}{\text{Var}\left[r_{t+1}^I\right]} \tag{36b}$$

$$\phi_j = \gamma^j \text{Var}_t\left[r_{X,t+1}^j\right] - \beta_j \text{Cov}\left[r_{t+1}^I, r_{j,t+1}^X\right] \tag{36c}$$

$$q_t^j = \frac{Y_t^j w_{X,j}^j}{Y_t^j} = \frac{Q_t^j}{Y_t^j} \tag{36d}$$

The segmentation variable in this case is a local variable, reflecting the market value of ineligible assets as a function of total wealth invested in that country (rather than total wealth invested worldwide).

The second difference with eligible assets is that the expected return on ineligible assets does not depend on the covariance with the global portfolio, but on all the individual covariances of country j's eligible assets with all the eligible markets in the world. The coefficients $\beta_j$result from the regression of the returns on ineligible assets $r_{j,t+1}^X$on all returns on eligible assets. In addition, the coefficients ϕ_j depend on the residualsε_{t+1} of this regression:

$$r_{i,t+1}^X = a_j + \beta_j r_{t+1}^I + \varepsilon_{j,t+1}$$

By substituting$\phi_j = \gamma_j \text{Var}\left[\varepsilon_{j,t+1}\right]$equation (3.36a) can be written as follows:

$$E\left[r_{i,t+1}^X\right] = \beta_j E_t\left[r_{t+1}^I\right] + \gamma_j \text{Var}\left[\varepsilon_{j,t+1}\right] q_t^j \tag{37}$$

This equation shows that in segmented markets, local variance is priced and local risk aversion determines the price of market risk.

Using a sample of 30 emerging markets grouped into 4 regions: Latin America, Asia and the Far East, Europe and the Middle East, and Africa, the authors calculated the mean and variance of the segmentation variable over the period January 1988-May 2000, which is based on the market value of eligible and ineligible assets in each country. Let's assume that V_t^j represents the value of assets in country j at time t that can be held by domestic and foreign investors, and that Q_t^j represents the value of assets in country j that can only be held by domestic investors. Total wealth invested in country j is therefore given by $Y_t^j = V_t^j + Q_t^j$. Consequently, the segmentation variable is defined by :

$$q_t^j = \frac{Q_t^j}{V_t^j + Q_t^j} = \frac{Q_t^j}{Y_t^j} \tag{38}$$

Empirical results show that there is some variation in the degree of segmentation in different countries. In some markets, such as Poland and South Africa, segmentation is low. Indeed, over 98% of assets can be freely traded by domestic and foreign investors. In other countries, such as Chile, China, India and Korea, more than 50% of assets are not accessible to foreign investors, showing that the degree of segmentation is high in these markets.

The standard deviations of the segmentation variable show a significant variation over time, confirming the findings of Bekaert and Harvey (1995) that the level of integration varies over time.

Jong and De Roon (2005) studied the effect of varying the degree of integration on the expected returns of emerging markets. q_t^j on expected returns in emerging markets and showed that expected returns in emerging markets are affected by the level of segmentation of the country itself, and by the level of segmentation of other countries in the region. In addition, expected returns in all four regions are affected by the level of segmentation of the region itself, and by the overall level of segmentation of emerging markets as a whole, as measured by the Emerging Markets Composite Index.

Tai (2007) examined the impact of the liberalization process on the cost of capital of emerging financial markets. Testing a conditional version of the CAPM International in the absence of PPP, over the period January 1986-April 2004, the author showed that the monthly risk premium of the Korean market fell from 1.14% to 0.503% after liberalization, a reduction of 56%. The cost of capital fell by 78% in the Philippines, 80% in Taiwan and 27% in Thailand.

V. FINANCIAL INTEGRATION TESTS

We showed in Chapter 1 that only systematic risk is remunerated by the market, so in a perfectly integrated international market only international systematic risk is remunerated, with variations from other sources considered residual. This is the starting assumption used by Solnik (1974) and Grauer, Litzenberger and Stehle (1976) in their International CAPM model.

In this world, the global market index is the optimal portfolio in a mean-variance plan. As a test of integration, it would be relatively easy to compose a global market portfolio and compare its return/variance ratios with those of individual market indices. This type of test would lead to the conclusion that financial markets are integrated, as the global market index would appear optimal. This conclusion would be erroneous, as it would presuppose the existence of an International CAPM where the return on financial assets is a function of the global market portfolio. However, studies have shown the difficulty of designing an International CAPM and validating it empirically. It is therefore necessary to distinguish between international CAPM tests and market integration tests. In this section, we want to know whether markets are integrated, i.e. whether the global market functions as a single market.

5.1 Financial integration tests based on CAPM

In the tests presented below, we will assume that the International CAPM is valid. The integration test then consists of empirically determining that the International CAPM provides a better asset valuation model than the domestic CAPM.

Solnik (1974) conducted a joint test of domestic CAPM and international CAPM on a sample of 234 stocks listed on the world's 9 largest markets between 1966-1971, to determine which model provided the best results. To do this, two equations are tested for each series of returns:

In the first equation, he regresses the return on each stock $R_{k,i}$in relation to the return of the market index $I_k$where it is quoted:

$$R_{k,i} = a_{k,i} + b_{k,i} I_k + \varepsilon_{k,i} \tag{39}$$

The average coefficient of determination (square of the correlation coefficient) obtained from these equations measures the proportion of the variance in a stock's return explained by variations in the market index.

According to the second equation, it regresses the return of each stock against the return of the global index. I_m :

$$R_{k,i} = a_{k,i} + b_{k,i}I_m + \varepsilon_{k,i} \tag{40}$$

Similarly, the correlation coefficient derived from this equation can be used to determine the proportion of each stock's variance explained by the global index.

The results show that national indices explain between 16% and 46% of variations in stock returns, while the global index explains only between 9% and 21%. So, although national factors are more influential, the international factor is not negligible.

However, Solnik's (1974) study comes up against a problem linked to the definition of a world stock market index. In fact, the calculation of this index[8] calls on several constraining assumptions. The exchange rates between the currencies in which the index returns are calculated are assumed to be stable over time. Investors in all the countries whose indices are used to calculate the global index have the same consumption baskets. Changes in individual preferences can lead to changes in real exchange rates. It would be necessary to modify the weighting of each index in the world index according to changes in individuals' consumption baskets, if the latter were to represent only fluctuations in securities returns.

The methodology used by Solnik (1974) assumes that the international factor and the national factor are totally independent, although the latter may have a common component which would explain some of the variations in the return on stock i in the first and second models. The integration test based on regression is therefore biased by the problem of collinearity between the international and national indices.

Stehle (1977) proposed an integration test that avoids this problem of collinearity between the domestic and international factors. He performed a domestic CAPM test and an international CAPM test on the same sample, isolating the component of the international factor whose variations are not explained by the domestic factor. To do this, he regressed the world stock market index $R_w$against the US stock market indexR_D.

$$R_w = a_{\mathrm{wD}} + \mathrm{b}R_D + v_w \tag{41}$$

The series of residual values $v_w$of the regression is therefore the component of the international factor not explained by the domestic factor. We can design a model based on the pure international factor, i.e. one that highlights for any stock i, a systematic international risk β_{iw} measured in relation to $v_w$the component of the international factor not explained by the domestic factor. The pure international beta$\beta_{\mathrm{iw}}$is calculated as follows:

$$\beta_{\mathrm{iw}} = \frac{\mathrm{Cov}(R_i, v_w)}{\mathrm{Var}(v_w)}$$

[8]This index was calculated by taking the weighted average of each index for the 9 countries considered, based on market capitalization.

We can then express the yield $R_i$as a function of the pure international factor and the national factor :

$$R_i = a_i + \beta_{i,d} R_d + \beta_{\mathrm{iw}} v_w + e_i \tag{42}$$

Where;

e_i A residual term.

Similarly, it is possible to isolate the component of the domestic factor that is not explained by the international factor. We can therefore express $R_i$as a function of the international factor and the pure domestic factor.

$$R_i = a'_i + \beta'_{i,w} R_w + \beta''_{\mathrm{id}} e'_d + u' \tag{43}$$

In this model, $\beta'_{i,w}$ provides a measure of i's total systematic risk in an international market and β''_{id} is the measure of risk that can be diversified internationally but not domestically.

Assuming that individuals have logarithmic utility functions, Stehle defines an international model of financial asset pricing where, in equilibrium, individuals hold portfolios that are optimal in terms of mean and variance, which can be written in two forms:

One where systematic risk is measured in relation to the national factor and the pure international factor:

$$E(R_i) = R_f + \beta_{i,d}\alpha_1 + \beta_{\mathrm{iw}}\alpha_2 \tag{44}$$

Where;

$\alpha_1 = E(R_i) - R_f$;

$\alpha_2 = \{\mathrm{Cov}(v_w, R_w - R_f)/\mathrm{Cov}\,(R_w, R_w - R_f)\}.[E(R_w) - R_f]$.

The other is expressed solely in terms of the international factor:

$$E(R_i) = R_f + \beta'_{\mathrm{iw}}[E(R_w) - R_f] \tag{45}$$

Similarly, the domestic CAPM can be written either as a function of the pure national factor, or as a function of the international factor. The market segmentation test then comes down to proving empirically whether the international factor α_2 is equal to zero. Similarly, the domestic CAPM can be written either as a function of the national factor, or as a function of the international factor and the pure national factor. In this model, the integration test amounts to proving whether the pure national factor parameter is equal to zero.

In his empirical test, Stehle calculated the world market index based on a sample of American, German, Belgian, Canadian, French, Japanese, Swiss, Dutch and British indices between January 1956 and December 1975. For the domestic market, the author used the US market. The results of the test do not allow us to reject or accept the market segmentation hypothesis.

Jorion and Schwartz (1986) used the same methodology as Stehle (1977), isolating the component of the international factor not explained by the domestic factor and the component of the domestic factor not explained by the international factor. They then demonstrate an International CAPM where, in equilibrium, individuals invest in a portfolio that is optimal in mean-variance space.

However, the originality of the study by Jorion and Schwartz (1986) lies in the fact that it is limited to a regional market, consisting of the United States and Canada. They examined the question of integration/segmentation of the Canadian market in relation to the overall North American market. In this study, integration is defined as a situation where investors obtain the same expected risk-adjusted return on the same financial instruments in different countries. With integration, the global market index should be mean-variance efficient, and consequently the only risk rewarded should be the systematic risk in relation to the global market. On the other hand, perfect segmentation implies that only national factors[9] are involved in the asset pricing relationship. The authors consider the two competing asset pricing models for valuing Canadian securities.

The international version of CAPM implies that :

$$E(R_i) = \gamma_0 + \gamma_1 \beta_i^G \tag{46}$$

Where;

$R_i = R_i^* - R_f$ The excess return on asset i is the difference between the nominal return and the risk-free rate. R^* and the risk-free rate ;

$R_G = R_G^* - R_f$: Excess yield on the global market ;

$R_C = R_C^* - R_f$: Excess returns on the Canadian market ;

β_i^G systematic risk in relation to the global market portfolio.

In accordance with equation (46), the systematic risk β_i^C.[10]relative to the Canadian portfolio $R_C$should have no explanatory power in asset pricing. However, as Stehle (1977) has shown, the integration hypothesis cannot be tested directly by running a univariate regression on β_i^Gbecause of the positive correlation between the Canadian and world markets. For this

[9] In other words, systematic domestic risk.

[10] β_i^C systematic risk in relation to the Canadian market portfolio.

reason, Jorion and Schwartz (1986) isolated the component of the domestic factor not explained by variations in the international index:

$$R_C = c_0 + c_1 R_G + V_{C.G}$$

The integration test must be based on the additional explanatory power of systematic risk $\beta_i^{C.G}$ (pure Canadian systematic risk) in relation to the residuals$V_{C.G}$. Consequently, the integration model can be reformulated as follows:

$$E(R_i) = \gamma_0 + \gamma_1 \beta_i^G + \gamma_2 \beta_i^{C.G} \qquad (47)$$

This is consistent with model (3.46) if the coefficient γ_2 is zero. An integration versus segmentation test, tests the null hypothesis that $\gamma_2 = 0$against the alternative hypothesis that $\gamma_2$is positive.

On the other hand, a segmented capital markets model assumes that expected returns $R_i$only remunerates systematic domestic risk:

$$E(R_i) = \delta_0 + \delta_1 \beta_i^C \qquad (48)$$

Similarly, by isolating the purely international component :

$$R_C = d_0 + d_1 R_C + V_{G.C}$$

And by calculating the beta of the asset $\beta_i^{G.C}$ (pure international systematic risk) relative to this residual, we obtain :

$$E(R_i) = \delta_0 + \delta_1 \beta_i^C + \delta_2 \beta_i^{G.C} \qquad (49)$$

Complete segmentation implies that $\delta_2 = 0$

To carry out the integration-segmentation test of the Canadian market vis-à-vis the overall North American market, the authors calculated monthly returns from January 1963 to December 1982 for stocks on the Toronto Stock Exchange for Canada and the New York Stock Exchange and American Stock Exchange for the USA. However, stocks listed simultaneously on both markets were isolated, to avoid double counting the same stocks. This is an important difference from the Stehle test, which did not take this precaution.

Using the maximum likelihood procedure, the empirical results show that γ_2 is significantly positive, rejecting the perfect integration hypothesis in favor of Canadian market segmentation. CAPM International is not the appropriate model for valuing Canadian assets over the 1963-1982 period. In fact, national factors, which are not present in the world index, are an important component of expected returns on Canadian securities.

Tai (2007) examined whether emerging markets became more integrated after liberalization, using a dynamic version of CAPM International in the absence of PPP (in the presence of exchange rate risk).

Starting from the conditional version of Errunza and Losq's (1985) model, which states that expected returns are a function of two risk factors, exposure to domestic market risk and global market risk, and introducing exchange rate risk based on the literature of Ferson and Harvey (1994), Dumas and Solnik (1995) and De Santis and Gerard (1998), Tai (2007) proposes the following model:

$$r_{i,t} = (1 - \mathrm{LD}_i)(\lambda_{w,t-1} h_{\mathrm{iw},t} + \lambda_{c,t-1} h_{\mathrm{ic},t}) + \mathrm{LD}_i \gamma_i h_{\mathrm{it}} + \varepsilon_{i,t}) \qquad \forall\, t \quad (50)$$

$$r_{w,t} = \lambda_{w,t-1} h_{w,t} + \lambda_{c,t-1} h_{c,t} + \varepsilon_{w,t}$$

$$r_{c,t} = \lambda_{w,t-1} h_{\mathrm{cw},t} + \lambda_{c,t-1} h_{c,t} + \varepsilon_{c,t}$$

Where;

$r_{w,t}$ Global market index excess return;

$r_{c,t}$ Exchange index performance;

$r_{i,t}$ The excess return on the market index for country i ;

$h_{i,t}$ The conditional variance of the market index for country i ;

$h_{w,t}$ The conditional variance of the world market index ;

$h_{c,t}$ The conditional variance of currency returns;

$h_{\mathrm{iw},t}$ The conditional covariance between the market index returns of country i and the world market index;

$h_{\mathrm{ic},t}$ The conditional covariance between the market index returns of country i and the exchange rate index;

$h_{\mathrm{cw},t}$ The conditional covariance between the returns of the world market index and the exchange rate index;

LD_i A liberalization dummy variable, equal to 1 before country i's liberalization date and 0 elsewhere.

The model stipulates that excess market returns in country i depend on country i-specific risk before liberalization, and on global market and exchange rate risks after liberalization. In the presence of this conditional CAPM, the market integration-segmentation test and the exchange rate risk assessment can be carried out jointly.

Using US dollar-denominated returns from 6 emerging market stock indices (India, Korea, Malaysia, Philippines, Taiwan and Thailand) and foreign exchange indices over the period January 1986-April 2004, and based on multivariate GARCH-in-Mean methodology, the results indicate that the Philippines was completely segmented prior to liberalization, whereas there was no evidence of perfect segmentation for the other five emerging markets, which were considered integrated. These results reinforce the role of exchange rate risk and the price of global market risk in explaining the dynamics of emerging market returns.

Hunter (2007) used ADRs to examine whether the emerging markets of Argentina, Chile and Mexico have become more integrated in the post-liberalization period. The author used an asset pricing model in which conditionally expected portfolio returns depend on the price of the US market's time varying risk and the exchange rate risk[11] . The null hypothesis of integration assumes equality between the risk price of the Latin American ADR portfolio and that of the US market portfolio. Consequently, deviation from zero in risk prices is synonymous with segmentation of emerging markets. The empirical results indicate that the markets examined did not become integrated after their liberalization, and this can be explained by the impact of currency crises on market segmentation.

5.2 Financial integration tests using CAPM Consumption

To test financial integration, several authors have used thc consumption-based asset pricing model of Stulz (1981a). In this model, the expected real return on an asset held by a representative investor is taken as a linear function of the covariance between its real return and the growth in its real consumption. Thus, the model predicts that there is an asset-pricing line for each country, which links the expected real return on the asset held by the representative investor to the covariance of this return with the growth of his real consumption.

5.2.1 CAPM consumption in the absence of barriers to international investment

The consumption CAPM assumes that deviations from power parity can arise from differences between the tastes of individuals in different countries, or from deviations from the law of one price. A representative investor will generally hold a portfolio that provides a hedge against changes in the prices of the goods consumed. If domestic assets are a more attractive means of hedging against changes in the price of the domestic consumption basket than foreign assets, then according to Stulz (1981a), the individual may choose a portfolio heavily weighted in domestic assets.

[11] The exchange rate index chosen in this equation is the US dollar price of the currencies of the 6 largest Latin American economies.

In this model, the expected real return in excess of the risk-free rate on an asset held by an individual is proportional to the covariance of this return with the growth in his real consumption :

$$\mu_{r_j^k} + \left(\sigma_{r_j^k}^2 2\right) = \Psi_k + \theta_k \sigma_{r_j^k, x_k} \tag{51}$$

Where;

$\mu_{r_j^k}(\sigma_{r_j^k}^2)$: The mean (variance) of the real return on j assets ;

Ψ_k Real return on risk-free assets;

θ_k The relative risk aversion of the representative investor in country k ;

x^k Growth in real individual consumption;

$\sigma_{r_j^k, x_k}$ The covariance between the real return on assets and the individual's real consumption.

5.2.2 CAPM Consumption and barriers to international investment

Wheatley (1988) has modeled barriers to international investment in a similar way to Stulz (1981b), i.e. barriers take the form of taxes on long and short positions of foreign assets.

This model assumes that asset j is located outside country k and that τ_j^k is a tax on the investor's long and short positions representing asset j belonging to country k . In the presence of this condition, foreign assets will not necessarily be located on the domestic valuation line (equation (51)):

$$\mu_{r_j^k} + \left(\sigma_{r_j^k}^2 2\right) = \pi_j^k + \Psi_k + \theta_k \sigma_{r_j^k, x_k} \tag{52}$$

Where ; $\pi_j^k = \tau_j^k(-\tau_j^k)$ if the individual has a long (short) position in asset j, whereas $-\tau_j^k \leq \pi_j^k \leq \tau_j^k$if the individual does not hold this asset.$|\pi_j^k|$ represents the distance between asset j and the domestic valuation line.

Wheatley's (1988) tests of the integration of international financial markets are conducted from the perspective of a US investor, using monthly data on the US market and 17 foreign markets[12] over the period December 1959-December 1985, and domestic data on real US consumption.

The author has attempted to test two hypotheses. The first hypothesis states that the expected real return on any U.S. asset is a linear function of its consumption beta, calculated

[12] Australia, Austria, Belgium, Canada, Denmark, France, Germany, Hong Kong, Italy, Japan, Netherlands, Norway, Singapore, Spain, Sweden, Switzerland and UK.

using actual U.S. consumption. The second hypothesis assumes that the expected real return on any US or non-US asset is a linear function of its consumption beta, calculated using real US consumption. The results show that the average real returns of US and non-US portfolios are positively related to their consumption betas. However, when calculating the distance between non-U.S. assets and the valuation line of U.S. domestic assets, the results indicate that foreign assets do not deviate significantly from the domestic line. Furthermore, due to the non-stationarity of the joint distribution of U.S. real consumption growth and real asset returns during the total 1959-1985 period (the distribution changed with the introduction of flexible exchange rates in March 1973), Wheatley (1988) tested the model for the two sub-periods: 1960-1973 and 1973-1985. The hypothesis that non-US portfolios do not move away from the domestic valuation line is also accepted in both sub-periods, showing that international capital markets are internationally integrated.

5.3 Determining the degree of market segmentation

Research results on international portfolio diversification have shown that investing in a market with a slightly segmented structure will result in abnormal returns for the international investor. Consequently, determining the degree of segmentation of a market in the rest of the world is of considerable importance. To this end, Akdogan (1996) proposed an approach for determining the degree of segmentation of financial markets in relation to world markets, using a fundamental instrument of modern portfolio theory à la Markowitz-Sharpe-Lintner, namely risk decomposition.

Consider the standard process that generates single-index returns:

$$R_i = \alpha_i + \beta_i R_w + \varepsilon_i$$

Where;

R_i The rate of return on the market portfolio of country i ;

R_w Global market rate of return ;

α_i The simple regression constant ;

β_i The beta of country i with respect to the market portfolio, $\beta_i = \frac{\mathrm{Cov}(R_i, R_w)}{\mathrm{Var}(R_w)}$.

The variance of the market portfolio of country i is determined as follows :

$$\mathrm{Var}(R_i) = \beta_i^2 \mathrm{Var}(R_w) + \mathrm{Var}(\varepsilon_i)$$

Dividing the two members of the equation by $\mathrm{Var}(R_i)$ we obtain :

$$p_i + q_i = 1$$

Where;

$$p_i = \frac{\beta_i^2 \mathrm{Var}(R_w)}{\mathrm{Var}(R_i)} \tag{53}$$

$$q_i = \frac{\mathrm{Var}(\varepsilon_i)}{\mathrm{Var}(R_i)} \tag{54}$$

The term p_i represents country i's share of systematic risk in the global portfolio, and measures this market's contribution to global market risk. Thus p_i is the measure of segmentation or integration of foreign market i into the global market. If p_i grows or alternatively q_i decreases over time, market i becomes more integrated into the global market and its contribution to international systematic risk decreases (and conversely if p_i decreases or q_i increases).

Using monthly data on 15 developed and 10 emerging markets, the author has estimated the evolution of these national markets' systematic risk shares in the world market (p_i) between 1972-1980 and 1981-1990. The results show that some markets became more integrated in the 1980s, such as the UK, Japan, France and Australia. The results also show that some European markets, such as Finland, Spain, Denmark and Italy, exhibit a slightly segmented structure, indicating that these markets are not perfectly segmented from the global market portfolio. However, although this study spans 19 years, it does not cover the recent period, and it is likely that some markets have changed their degree of integration into the global market.

In a more recent study, Barari (2004) extended Akdogan's (1996) approach to measure the degree of integration of national markets in relation to two market portfolios: the global index and the regional index. This procedure makes it possible to compare the importance of regional integration with that of global integration.

In this model, the two-index return-generating process for the domestic market portfolio i is as follows:

$$R_i = \alpha_i + \beta_{\mathrm{ir}} U_r + \beta_{\mathrm{iw}} R_w + \varepsilon_i \tag{55}$$

Where;

β_{iw} The beta of market index i relative to the global benchmark ;

β_{ir} The beta of market index i relative to the regional benchmark ;

ε_i A random error term ;

R_w The rate of return of the global index.

U_r The residual of the following regression :

$$R_r = \alpha_r + \beta_r R_w + U_r \tag{56}$$

Where;

R_r The rate of return on the regional index.

In equation (56), $U_r$represents the part of the variation in $R_r$that is not explained by R_w(which is therefore orthogonal toR_w). By taking the variance of the two members of equation (55) and dividing by$\text{var}(R_i)$the risk associated with the portfolio of country i is decomposed as follows:

$$a_i + b_i + c_i = 1$$

Where;

$$a_i = \frac{\beta_{\text{ir}}^2 \text{var}(U_r)}{\text{var}(R_i)} \tag{57}$$

$$b_i = \frac{\beta_{\text{iw}}^2 \text{var}(R_w)}{\text{var}(R_i)} \tag{58}$$

$$c_i = \frac{\text{var}(\varepsilon_i)}{\text{var}(R_i)} \tag{59}$$

a_i measures country i's contribution to regional systematic risk (which is uncorrelated with global systematic risk), $b_i$measures country i's contribution to global systematic risk, and $c_i$measures country i's unsystematic risk.

By dividing the degrees of integration a_i and $b_i$by their relative shares in regional and global market capitalization[13] , we obtain the adjusted degrees of integration:

$$a_i \text{ ajusté} = \frac{a_i}{W_r}$$

$$b_i \text{ ajusté} = \frac{b_i}{W_w}$$

$$W_r = \frac{\text{MC}_i}{\sum_{i=1}^{n} \text{MC}_i}$$

$$W_w = \frac{\text{MC}_i}{\sum_{i=1}^{m} \text{MC}_i}$$

Where;

MC: market capitalization ;

m: number of countries in the global index ;

n: number of countries in the regional index.

[13] Since market capitalizations vary over time, the author has divided the share of systematic risk by the share of market capitalization in the region and worldwide.

To examine the variation over time in the degree of global and regional integration of 6 countries in the Latin American region[14] , Barari (2004) employed a time-varying approach based on historical prices and the moving average. The results indicate that Latin American countries are more regionally integrated and less internationally integrated in the late eighties and early nineties. However, from the mid-nineties onwards, these countries became more globally integrated with the developed countries and emerging markets of other regions, mainly after the Asian crisis, with the exception of Venezuela and Colombia, where regional and global integration is very weak. This can be partly attributed to the political instability of these countries during the study period.

The author also calculated the ratio between the degree of regional integration and the degree of global integration[15] . All countries show an increasing trend in the ratio $\frac{a}{b}$ until the mid-90s, suggesting that regional integration is more important than global integration. At the end of the 90s, this ratio became decreasing, showing the trend of countries towards global integration.

5.4 Tests based on the Cointegration technique

Several studies have measured the integration of financial markets by identifying common long-term stochastic trends using the cointegration method. Allen and MacDonald (1995) studied the links between Asian markets and confirmed their segmentations. Piesse and Hearn (2002) examined the question of integration from January 1990 to January 2000 for the three largest markets in South African countries: Botswana, Namibia and South Africa. The results of the cointegration analysis indicate that there is a cointegrating vector in the bivariate VAR system between South Africa and Namibia that is common to the underlying stochastic data series, indicating the existence of a long-term structural relationship. For the other country pairs, Namibia-Botswana and South Africa-Botswana, the results show no long-term relationship. The results of Granger causality tests indicate that causality is unidirectional from Namibia to South Africa. Indeed, South Africa's market is larger than Namibia's in terms of market capitalization, has greater access to international capital markets and could therefore be less influenced by a local or regional factor than Namibia.

Aloui and Bouanani (2005) examined the degree of integration of Middle Eastern and North African (MENA) countries using a bi- and multivariate cointegration approach. The empirical study was carried out on a sample of nine Arab countries[16] and three world stock

[14] Argentina, Brazil, Chile, Colombia, Mexico and Venezuela.

[15] The ratio $\frac{a}{b}$.

[16] Tunisia, Morocco, Egypt, Jordan, Oman, Saudi Arabia, Lebanon, Kuwait and Bahrain.

exchanges over the period 1996-2003. The results show that MENA stock markets are highly segmented. Indeed, cointegration tests show the absence of a stable long-term equilibrium between the different Arab stock exchanges. In fact, only one cointegrating relationship was detected between the Kuwait and Bahrain stock exchanges. This relationship can be explained by the free-trade agreements between these two oil-producing countries and their membership of the Gulf Cooperation Council. With regard to the integration of MENA markets with certain international financial markets, the results show the integration of certain Arab stock exchanges with those of Germany, France and the United States.

Davies (2006) examined the issue of international financial market integration using several cointegration techniques. Based on Engle and Granger's (1987) and Johansen's (1988,1994) approach, the author rejected cointegration between the global index and any of the following markets: Australia, Canada, Germany, Japan, Switzerland, the UK and the USA. These results can be explained by the presence of multiple structural breaks. Davies (2006) also estimated the residual terms of the long-term relationship, based on the Markov change estimate introduced by Hamilton (1990). This analysis assumes the presence of multiple changes in the long-term relationship. The test results indicate the existence of stationary residual series in all long-term relationships, supporting the integration of developed markets into the global market in the presence of regime shifts.

VI. THE WORLD PRICE OF COVARIANCE RISK: TESTING CONDITIONAL VERSIONS OF CAPM INTERNATIONAL

Studies examining the international version of the CAPM are numerous. Tests of Sharpe's (1964) and Lintner's (1965) Asset Pricing Model have been carried out by Solnik (1974, 1977), Stehle (1977), Stulz (1984) etc. Multifactor Asset Pricing Models have been tested by Cho, Eun and Senbet (1986), Hamao (1988), Gultekin, Gultekin and Penati (1989) and Korajczyk and Viallet (1989). Wheatley (1988) tested the Asset Valuation Model on an international scale, based on consumption. All these studies evaluated only the unconditional moments inferred by the models. They therefore sought to explain whether cross-sectional differences in risk explain differences in average returns. Our study focuses on the conditional valuation of financial assets on an international scale.

The aim of this chapter is to verify the ability of the conditional versions of Sharpe's (1964) and Lintner's (1965) Asset Pricing Model to explain the behavior of stock market returns in 22 countries, and to test the mean-variance efficiency of the world market portfolio.

Based on the work of Harvey (1991), country risk is defined as the conditional sensitivity (covariance) of a country's stock market performance to world stock market performance. This risk is subject to variations over time. The remuneration per unit of sensitivity is the world price of covariance risk. We will proceed as follows:

First, we will present measures of the conditional moments of the financial returns of individual countries and of the return on the global financial market.

Secondly, we will calculate the conditional covariances in the different countries and check whether they explain the dynamic behavior of stock market returns.

Thirdly, we'll calculate the global price of covariance risk in different countries and see if it's constant in the world's 7 largest countries.

6.1 Presentation of test models

6.1.1 CAPM International with time-varying moments

The conditional version of the Asset Pricing Model by Sharpe (1964) and Lintner (1965), assumes that the conditionally expected return on an asset is proportional to its covariance with the market portfolio. The weighting factor is the price of covariance risk, i.e. the remuneration (expected return) obtained by the investor for taking one unit of covariance risk. The model is as follows:

$$E\left[r_{jt} | \Omega_{t-1}\right] = \frac{E[r_{mt} | \Omega_{t-1}]}{\mathrm{Var}[r_{mt} | \Omega_{t-1}]} \mathrm{Cov}\left[r_{jt}, r_{mt} | \Omega_{t-1}\right] \tag{60}$$

Where;

r_{jt} the return on the market portfolio of country j between t and t-1, in excess of the risk-free rate ;

r_{mt} excess return on the global market portfolio ;

Ω_{t-1} The set of information used by investors to evaluate asset prices;

$E\left[r_{mt} | \Omega_{t-1}\right]$ The conditionally expected return on the world market ;

$\mathrm{Var}[r_{mt} | \Omega_{t-1}]$ The conditional variance of the world market ;

The ratio $\frac{E[r_{mt} | \Omega_{t-1}]}{\mathrm{Var}[r_{mt} | \Omega_{t-1}]}$ is the world price of covariance risk.

To test equation (60), we will follow Harvey's (1991) methodology. To do this, we'll assume that investors only have access to a subset of informationZ_{t-1}In this case, the forecast error is equal to the difference between the realized return and the expected return:

$$u_{jt} = r_{jt} - Z_{t-1}\delta_j \tag{61}$$

Where;

u_{jt} investor's forecast error for country j's return ;

Z_{t-1} : l variables of information available to the investor ;

δ_j a set of coefficients used by the investor to derive conditionally expected returns.

Equation (60) can then be expressed as follows:

$$Z_{t-1}\delta_j = \frac{Z_{t-1}\delta_m}{E\left[u_{mt}^2 | Z_{t-1}\right]} E\left[u_{jt}u_{mt} | Z_{t-1}\right] \tag{62}$$

Where;

u_{mt} The investor's forecast error for the return on the world market portfolio.

Note that $E\left[u_{mt}^2 | Z_{t-1}\right]$ is the conditional variance (of the forecast error) and $E\left[u_{jt}u_{mt} | Z_{t-1}\right]$ is the conditional covariance. Multiplying this equation by the conditional variance gives :

$$E\left[u_{mt}^2 Z_{t-1}\delta_j | Z_{t-1}\right] = E\left[u_{jt}u_{mt}Z_{t-1}\delta_m | Z_{t-1}\right] \tag{63}$$

The deviation from expectations is :

$$h_{jt} = u_{mt}^2 Z_{t-1}\delta_j - u_{jt}u_{mt}Z_{t-1}\delta_m \tag{64}$$

Where;

h_{jt} error: the error that is unrelated to the information, in the presence of the null hypothesis that the model is verified.

If the error $h_{jt}$is divided by the conditional variance of the world market return, it can be interpreted as the deviation of the country's return from the return predicted by the model ($h_{jt}$is the valuation error). If $h_{jt}$is positive, this implies that the model is undervaluing country j's performance; if $h_{jt}$is negative, the CAPM is overvaluing stock market returns.

The econometric model to be tested is formed by combining equations (61) and (64) :

$$\varepsilon_t = (u_t u_{\mathrm{mt}} h_t) = \begin{pmatrix} [r_t - Z_{t-1}\delta]' \\ [r_{\mathrm{mt}} - Z_{t-1}\delta_m]' \\ [u_{\mathrm{mt}}^2 Z_{t-1}\delta - u_{\mathrm{mt}} u_t Z_{t-1}\delta_m]' \end{pmatrix} \quad (65)$$

Where;

u This vector is of dimension (1 x n), where n is the number of countries.

The model implies that $E[\varepsilon_t|Z_{t-1}] = 0$. With n countries, there are n+1 columns of disturbances at the conditional mean level (u and u_m) and n columns in$h$.

To estimate the parameters of equation (65), we'll use Hansen's (1982) generalized method of moments (GMM). Since the model presents $l$information variables, there will be $[l \times (2n + 1)]$ orthogonality conditions, $[l \times (n + 1)]$parameters to be estimated and consequently, $l \times n$over-identification conditions.

6.1.2 The global price of covariance risk

In equation (65), all conditional moments, i.e. means, variances and covariances, are assumed to be time-varying. If one of the moments is constant, other versions of the model can be obtained.

Traditionally, asset valuation tests assume that expected returns are proportional to the expected return of a benchmark portfolio.

This hypothesis can be tested as follows:

$$k_t = r_t - r_{\mathrm{mt}}\beta \quad (66)$$

Where;

β A vector of n volatility coefficients, it represents the ratios of the conditional covariances of the excess returns of the various countries to the conditional variance of the benchmark return.

The model implies that$E[k_t|Z_{t-1}] = 0$where k_t is the evaluation error associated with this model. There are $l \times n$ orthogonality conditions and n parameters to estimate, leading to $[n \times (l-1)]$ over-identification conditions to be tested.

Another version of the model assumes that the remuneration of the volatility ratio is constant. In this model, this remuneration is the world price of covariance risk. By imposing this constraint, the valuation error associated with the assumption that the price of covariance risk is constant :

$$e_t = r_t - \lambda u_t u_{\mathrm{mt}} \tag{67}$$

Where;

λ The ratio of the conditionally expected market return divided by the conditional covariance ;

e_t Valuation error associated with the assumption of a constant price of covariance risk.

The model for equation (67) is as follows:

$$\varepsilon_t = (u_t u_{\mathrm{mt}} e_t) = \begin{pmatrix} [r_t - Z_{t-1}\delta]' \\ [r_{\mathrm{mt}} - Z_{t-1}\delta_m]' \\ [r_t - \lambda(u_{\mathrm{mt}} u_t)]' \end{pmatrix} \tag{68}$$

With n assets, there are n+1 columns in $u$and $u_m$and n columns in e.

To simplify the estimation of the system of equations (68), we consider that $E[u_{\mathrm{mt}} u_{\mathrm{jt}}|Z_{t-1}] = E[u_{\mathrm{mt}} r_{\mathrm{jt}}|Z_{t-1}]$.[17]. A simpler system is therefore estimated :

$$\eta_t = (u_{\mathrm{mt}} e_t) = \begin{pmatrix} [r_{\mathrm{mt}} - Z_{t-1}\delta_m]' \\ [r_t - \lambda(u_{\mathrm{mt}} r_t)]' \end{pmatrix} \tag{69}$$

This system has n+1 equations and $[l \times (n+1)]$ orthogonality conditions. With $l+1$ parameters, there are $(l \times n) - 1$over-identification conditions to test.

6.2 Data description and choice of instrumental variables

The study is conducted from the perspective of an American investor. Returns are therefore calculated in US dollars. The yield on the 30-day U.S. Treasury note is the

---

17
$$\begin{aligned} E[u_{\mathrm{mt}} u_{\mathrm{jt}}|Z_{t-1}] &= E[u_{\mathrm{mt}}(r_{\mathrm{jt}} - Z_{t-1}\delta_j)|Z_{t-1}] \\ &= E[u_{\mathrm{mt}} r_{\mathrm{jt}}|Z_{t-1}] - E[u_{\mathrm{mt}} Z_{t-1}\delta_j|Z_{t-1}] \\ &= E[u_{\mathrm{mt}} r_{\mathrm{jt}}|Z_{t-1}] - E[u_{\mathrm{mt}}|Z_{t-1}]Z_{t-1}\delta_j \\ &= E[u_{\mathrm{mt}} r_{\mathrm{jt}}|Z_{t-1}] \end{aligned}$$

Since $E[u_{\mathrm{mt}}|Z_{t-1}] = 0$

conditionally risk-free yield. All returns are calculated in excess of the yield on the U.S. Treasury bond.

The data used in this study are the global index, the global emerging markets index and the stock market indices of 15 developed financial markets and 7 emerging markets[18] . All data are monthly and come from Morgan Stanley Capital International. The observation period runs from December 1987 to December 2004, for a total of 205 observations.

Since stock market returns are assumed to be time-varying, it is necessary to introduce instrumental variables to predict stock market returns. These instrumental variables should approximate the information used by investors to value financial assets.

In line with Harvey (1991) and Bekaert and Harvey (1995), we will use two sets of instrumental variables: instruments common to all countries, and country-specific local instruments.

The global information variables are made up of the excess lagged yield of the global market, a dummy variable for the month of January, the change in the forward structure of the US market, and the US default risk spread.

Indeed, previous empirical work shows that stock market returns exhibit a certain degree of autocorrelation, which explains the introduction of lagged returns among the instrumental variables. In addition, Keim (1983) has shown that US returns are systematically higher in January. Similarly, Gultekin and Gultekin (1983) demonstrated the existence of a January effect in several industrialized countries. Keim and Stambaugh (1986) and Fama and French (1989) showed that the U.S. default risk spread, measured by the difference between Moody's Baa and Aaa bond yields, helps predict yields. Campbell and Hamao (1992) highlighted the effect of term structure on financial returns in the US and Japan. Consequently, the excess return on the 3-month Treasury bill was used as a common instrumental variable.

Local instrumental variables consist of country-specific lagged stock market returns. The choice of instrumental variables is limited by the availability of data, which comes from Economagic Data.

[18] United States, Germany, Australia, Austria, Belgium, Canada, Spain, France, Hong Kong, Italy, Japan, Netherlands, United Kingdom, Sweden, Switzerland (15 developed markets), Argentina, Chile, Korea, Indonesia, Malaysia, Mexico and Thailand (7 emerging markets)

6.3 Descriptive statistics for stock market returns

Table (1) shows averages and standard deviations over the period 1987-2004 for developed and emerging markets. The analysis is based on monthly MSCI index returns expressed in US dollars, in excess of the 1-month US Treasury bill. The average excess return for developed countries ranges from -0.02% (Japan) to 1.1% (Sweden), while the average return for emerging countries ranges from 0.67% (Malaysia) to 2.3% (Argentina). In fact, with the exception of Korea, Malaysia and Thailand, yields in developing countries are higher than in developed markets. What's more, emerging markets are much more volatile than industrialized markets. As a result, investment in emerging markets is characterized by a fairly high Markowitz risk-return trade-off.

We also note that the USA has the lowest volatility. In fact, the American market dominates the whole world in terms of risk minimization. This is in line with Harvey's (1991) analysis of the 1969-1989 period and that of Bekaert and Harvey (1995).

It's worth noting that the level of risk in the US market is similar to that of the global market portfolio, which is the value-weighted average of the stock market returns of the various countries. For a risk-averse investor, investing in either the world market or the US market provides the lowest standard deviation.

This result is not surprising, given that the US market occupies a significant share of the world market. What's more, most US firms listed on the financial markets are multinationals, which is reflected in the high level of correlation between the US market and the world market (0.83).

Table (1): Descriptive statistics for excess returns on financial markets: (1987:12-2004:12)

Developed markets		**Average**	**Standard deviation**
Germany	ALL	0.0070	0.0646
Australia	AUS	0.0059	0.0539
Austria	AT	0.0074	0.0664
Belgium	BEL	0.0068	0.0524
Canada	CAN	0.0060	0.0502
Spain	ESP	0.0068	0.0637
United States	USA	0.0072	0.0414
France	FR	0.0079	0.0571
Hong Kong	HK	0.0092	0.0795
Italy	IT	0.0053	0.0684
Japan	JP	-0.0002	0.0679
Netherlands	PB	0.0065	0.0491
United Kingdom	RU	0.0048	0.0462
Sweden	SUE	0.0110	0.0741
Switzerland	SUI	0.0085	0.0502
Global index	**World**	**0.0045**	**0.0414**

Emerging markets		**Average**	**Standard deviation**
Argentina	ARG	0.0231	0.1706
Chile	CHI	0.0125	0.0733
Korea	COR	0.0083	0.1181
Indonesia	IND	0.0141	0.1606
Malaysia	MAL	0.0067	0.0937
Mexico	MEX	0.0196	0.0974
Thailand	THA	0.0083	0.1208
Global Emerging Markets Index	**EM**	**0.0091**	**0.0669**

Similarly, as a number of researchers have shown, it is worth investing in emerging markets when their correlation with other markets is low, thereby reducing overall portfolio risk. Table (2) shows the correlation matrix between the various markets.

Table (2): Yield correlation matrix (1987:01-2004:12)

	EM	WD	THA	MEX	MAL	IND	COR	CHI	ARG	SUI	SUE	RU	PB	JP	IT	HK	FR	USA	ESP	CAN	BEL	AT	AUS	ALL
ALL	0.46	0.71	0.31	0.32	0.31	0.18	0.20	0.27	0.08	0.61	0.69	0.64	0.81	0.30	0.59	0.39	0.81	0.58	0.64	0.52	0.69	0.56	0.43	1.00
AUS	0.53	0.58	0.46	0.37	0.28	0.25	0.38	0.28	0.25	0.36	0.52	0.55	0.50	0.38	0.30	0.46	0.44	0.49	0.50	0.59	0.31	0.29	1.00	0.43
AT	0.38	0.37	0.27	0.19	0.31	0.29	0.12	0.19	0.10	0.48	0.31	0.45	0.50	0.23	0.39	0.32	0.45	0.21	0.41	0.29	0.43	1.00	0.29	0.56
BEL	0.32	0.63	0.25	0.24	0.17	0.16	0.18	0.19	0.06	0.61	0.44	0.58	0.73	0.31	0.48	0.29	0.71	0.50	0.55	0.38	1.00	0.43	0.31	0.69
CAN	0.59	0.72	0.43	0.44	0.41	0.32	0.32	0.39	0.20	0.44	0.58	0.52	0.57	0.38	0.43	0.57	0.53	0.74	0.50	1.00	0.38	0.29	0.59	0.52
ESP	0.56	0.73	0.31	0.40	0.28	0.18	0.27	0.33	0.23	0.56	0.70	0.63	0.66	0.44	0.60	0.43	0.66	0.56	1.00	0.50	0.55	0.41	0.50	0.64
USA	0.58	0.83	0.43	0.48	0.32	0.24	0.34	0.39	0.21	0.52	0.61	0.64	0.66	0.34	0.38	0.49	0.60	1.00	0.56	0.74	0.50	0.21	0.49	0.58
FR	0.45	0.74	0.26	0.34	0.27	0.18	0.21	0.24	0.19	0.64	0.63	0.66	0.78	0.38	0.56	0.39	1.00	0.60	0.66	0.53	0.71	0.45	0.44	0.81
HK	0.65	0.55	0.54	0.41	0.55	0.35	0.29	0.43	0.18	0.33	0.43	0.47	0.45	0.33	0.26	1.00	0.39	0.49	0.43	0.57	0.29	0.32	0.46	0.39
IT	0.36	0.56	0.22	0.26	0.20	0.17	0.23	0.24	0.07	0.44	0.53	0.44	0.55	0.33	1.00	0.26	0.56	0.38	0.60	0.43	0.48	0.39	0.30	0.59
JP	0.39	0.71	0.30	0.23	0.23	0.12	0.44	0.13	-.005	0.43	0.42	0.46	0.41	1.00	0.33	0.33	0.38	0.34	0.44	0.38	0.31	0.23	0.38	0.30
PB	0.49	0.79	0.31	0.29	0.36	0.21	0.25	0.28	0.10	0.72	0.67	0.75	1.00	0.41	0.55	0.45	0.78	0.66	0.66	0.57	0.73	0.50	0.50	0.81
RU	0.44	0.80	0.28	0.30	0.31	0.12	0.29	0.24	0.08	0.66	0.60	1.00	0.75	0.46	0.44	0.47	0.66	0.64	0.63	0.52	0.58	0.45	0.55	0.64
SUE	0.56	0.75	0.30	0.36	0.34	0.21	0.32	0.32	0.13	0.53	1.00	0.60	0.67	0.42	0.53	0.43	0.63	0.61	0.70	0.58	0.44	0.31	0.52	0.69
SUI	0.37	0.68	0.27	0.23	0.25	0.20	0.22	0.20	.002	1.00	0.53	0.66	0.72	0.43	0.44	0.33	0.64	0.52	0.56	0.44	0.61	0.48	0.36	0.61
ARG	0.35	0.13	0.17	0.38	0.12	0.14	0.05	0.24	1.00	0.00	0.13	0.08	0.10	-.005	0.07	0.18	0.19	0.21	0.23	0.20	0.06	0.10	0.25	0.08
CHI	0.60	0.34	0.37	0.37	0.34	0.24	0.23	1.00	0.24	0.20	0.32	0.24	0.28	0.13	0.24	0.43	0.24	0.39	0.33	0.39	0.19	0.19	0.28	0.27
COR	0.40	0.43	0.48	0.25	0.28	0.29	1.00	0.23	0.05	0.22	0.32	0.29	0.25	0.44	0.23	0.29	0.21	0.34	0.27	0.32	0.18	0.12	0.38	0.20
IND	0.38	0.21	0.41	0.22	0.42	1.00	0.29	0.24	0.14	0.20	0.21	0.12	0.21	0.12	0.17	0.35	0.18	0.24	0.18	0.32	0.16	0.29	0.25	0.18
MAL	0.58	0.39	0.53	0.27	1.00	0.42	0.28	0.34	0.12	0.25	0.34	0.31	0.36	0.23	0.20	0.55	0.27	0.32	0.28	0.41	0.17	0.31	0.28	0.31
MEX	0.63	0.45	0.36	1.00	0.27	0.22	0.25	0.37	0.38	0.23	0.36	0.30	0.29	0.23	0.26	0.41	0.34	0.48	0.40	0.44	0.24	0.19	0.37	0.32
THA	0.59	0.43	1.00	0.36	0.53	0.41	0.48	0.37	0.17	0.27	0.30	0.28	0.31	0.30	0.22	0.54	0.26	0.43	0.31	0.43	0.25	0.27	0.46	0.31
WD	0.63	1.00	0.43	0.45	0.39	0.21	0.43	0.34	0.13	0.68	0.75	0.80	0.79	0.71	0.56	0.55	0.74	0.83	0.73	0.72	0.63	0.37	0.58	0.71
EM	1.00	0.63	0.59	0.63	0.58	0.38	0.40	0.60	0.35	0.37	0.56	0.44	0.49	0.39	0.36	0.65	0.45	0.58	0.56	0.59	0.32	0.38	0.53	0.46

The correlation of emerging market returns with developed markets and with the world market is very low, and even negative for some countries such as Argentina. The correlation between developed markets and the world index ranges from 0.37 (Austria) to 0.83 (USA), while it varies from 0.13 (Argentina) to 0.45 (Mexico) for emerging markets. These results are not surprising, given that the Mexican market is currently one of the most capitalized (US$ 171402 million at the end of 2004[19]) in the world. It became fully open to foreign investors in 1989. Argentina had a market capitalization of US$40593 million in 2004. In conclusion, the results demonstrate the importance of developing countries for an international portfolio.

Table (3): Simple autocorrelation functions for stock market returns

Developed markets		ρ_1	ρ_2	ρ_3	ρ_4	ρ_{12}
Germany	ALL	-0.062	-0.031	0.012	-0.009	0.035
Australia	AUS	-0.069	0.005	-0.011	-0.174*	0.021
Austria	AT	0.098	-0.045	-0.046	0.142*	-0.033
Belgium	BEL	0.068	0.006	-0.136	-0.020	0.020
Canada	CAN	0.087	-0.030	0.065	-0.090	-0.085
Spain	ESP	-0.017	-0.106	0.018	-0.052	-0.051
United States	USA	-0.043	-0.019	0.057	-0.064	0.038
France	FR	0.075	-0.089	0.034	-0.016	-0.022
Hong Kong	HK	0.055	-0.045	-0.084	-0.097	-0.082
Italy	IT	-0.116	-0.056	0.040	0.042	0.118
Japan	JP	0.020	-0.038	0.092	-0.066	-0.046
Netherlands	PB	-0. 109	-0.011	-0.050	-0.052	0.106
United Kingdom	RU	-0.032	-0.168	-0.087	0.024	0.005
Sweden	SUE	0.035	-0.060	0.079	-0.050	-0.022
Switzerland	SUI	0.042	-0.129	-0.036	-0.104	0.017

* indicates statistics that are significantly different from zero at the 5% level.

$t^{\alpha/2}\frac{1}{\sqrt{n}}$=1,96*1$\sqrt{204}$=0,1372.

[19] According to the World Federation of Stock Exchanges.

Emerging markets		ρ_1	ρ_2	ρ_3	ρ_4	ρ_{12}
Argentina	ARG	0.056	-0.056	-0.025	0.087	0.066
Chile	CHI	0.176*	-0.029	-0.058	0.049	0.067
Korea	COR	0.014	-0.015	0.008	-0.071	-0.076
Indonesia	IND	0.129	-0.070	-0.039	0.071	-0.051
Malaysia	MAL	0.125	0.204*	-0.083	-0.037	0.015
Mexico	MEX	0.076	0.003	0.030	-0.080	0.012
Thailand	THA	0.038	0.140	-0.088	-0.166*	0.085
Global index	World	-0.017	-0.062	0.005	-0.086	0.046
Overall ME index	EM	0.174*	0.057	-0.019	-0.146*	0.042

* indicates statistics that are significantly different from zero at the 5% level.
$t^{\alpha/2}\frac{1}{\sqrt{n}}$=1,96*1√204=0,1372.

The study of simple autocorrelation functions indicates that, with the exception of Australia and Austria, the first-order autocorrelations of developed market returns are not significant. Emerging market returns are more autocorrelated than developed markets. Argentina, Chile, Malaysia and the overall emerging market portfolio exhibit high autocorrelations.

6.4 Empirical results

6.4.1 Conditional CAPM test with time-varying moments

We began our empirical analysis by estimating the system of equations (65), i.e. the general model that allows expected returns, variances and covariances to vary instantaneously. The test was carried out individually for each country and for the G7 as a whole (table (4)).

The statistic forχ^2statistic, known as the overidentification test or J-statistic, has a degree of freedom equal to the number of orthogonality conditions minus the number of parameters to be estimated. This statistic examines the null hypothesis that the global market portfolio is conditionally efficient in the sense of mean-variance[20] .

The $\overline{R^2}$statistic represents the adjusted coefficient of determination of a regression of model errors on global information variables. If the model is well specified, the errors would be unrelated to the information and$\chi^2$and $\overline{R^2}$would be small.

[20] A high χ^2indicates that the errors are correlated with the instrumental variables.

The asset pricing model for individual countries tests the hypothesis that a country's conditionally expected return is proportional to its covariance with world returns. For the G7 countries as a whole, the model tests the hypothesis that the global price of covariance risk[21] is constant in the world's 7 largest countries.

Test results for individual countries with global variables indicate that the model's hypotheses are rejected at the 5% significance level for 7 developed countries: Australia, Belgium, Canada, Hong Kong, Japan, Netherlands and Switzerland. With local variables, the hypotheses are validated for Canada and Switzerland.

The results of individual tests carried out on emerging markets also depend on the choice of information variables. With global instruments, the hypothesis of global market portfolio efficiency is validated at the 5% significance level for only two countries: Argentina and Malaysia. With local instruments, the null hypothesis of world market efficiency became valid for 4 countries (Argentina, Korea, Malaysia and Indonesia).

For all the G7, the model's hypotheses are not rejected at the standard significance level. Using local or global information variables, the global portfolio is conditionally efficient in the mean-variance sense.

The table shows further information on valuation errors, based on estimates with common instrumental variables. Positive errors are found for Austria, Italy and the Netherlands, (for the group of developed countries), Korea, Indonesia, Mexico and Thailand (for the group of emerging markets), indicating that, given the level of risk, the actual return is on average higher than the expected return, and vice versa for the negative valuation error. Likewise, it is important to note that the USA recorded the lowest average error over the 1987-2004 period.

We also note that the ranking of average conditional covariances is different from that of average yields. However, it is interesting to show that Sweden has the highest average conditional covariance, as well as the highest average yield.

[21]the world price of covariance risk is the conditionally expected return on the world market divided by the conditional variance.

Table (4): Estimation of conditional CAPM with instantaneous expected returns, variances and covariances

Developed Markets	Average yield	Covariance conditional average	Average error	$\overline{R^2}$	Instruments global : Statistics J (*P-value*)	Local instruments : Statistics J (*P-value*)
Germany	0.0070	1.968	-0.00023	-0.0119	0.039426 (0.0914)	0.0346 (0.1337)
Australia	0.0059	1.322	-0.0082	0.0858	0.073408 (0.0049)	0.0601 (0.0158)
Austria	0.0074	1.073	0.003448	0.0187	0.042111 (0.0734)	0.0209 (0.3724)
Belgium	0.0068	1.416	-0.03190	-0.0050	0.048602 (0.0427)	0.0556 (0.0234)
Canada	0.0060	1.519	-0.04153	0.0992	0.057916 (0.0192)	0.0454 (0.0558)
Spain	0.0060	1.949	-0.00055	-0.0144	0.019199 (0.420)	0.0154 (0.534)
United States	0.0072	1.453	0.000430	-0.0125	0.044054 (0.0625)	0.0448 (0.0587)
France	0.0068	1.79	-7.55E-05	-0.0034	0.031799 (0.1676)	0.0339 (0.1419)
Hong Kong	0.0092	1.889	-0.00025	-0.0140	0.049554 (0.0394)	0.0487 (0.0422)
Italy	0.0053	1.614	0.001289	-0.0142	0.024369 (0.292)	0.0341 (0.139)
Japan	-0.0002	2.00	-0.00349	-0.0101	0.049014 (0.0412)	0.0489 (0.0414)
Netherlands	0.0065	1.642	0.000374	-0.0093	0.073870 (0.0047)	0.0695 (0.0069)
United Kingdom	0.0048	1.558	-0.01082	-0.0096	0.026026 (0.256)	0.0320 (0.1643)
Sweden	0.0110	2.321	0.007299	-0.0109	0.042929 (0.0686)	0.0299 (0.1939)
Switzerland	0.0085	1.462	-0.00468	-0.0102	0.051176 (0.0343)	0.0424 (0.0716)
G7					0.125419 (0.6026)	0.1566 (0.2826)

Emerging markets	Average yield	Covariance conditional average	Average error	$\overline{R^2}$	Instruments global : Statistics J (*P-value*)	Local instruments : Statistics J (*P-value*)
Argentina	0.0231	1.100	-0.01331	-0.0128	0.03658 (0.114)	0.0340 (0.1409)
Chile	0.0125	1.048	-0.00523	-0.0085	0.058048 (0.0190)	0.0556 (0.0234)
Korea	0.0083	2.099	0.010102	0.0176	0.047972 (0.0450)	0.0333 (0.1483)
Indonesia	0.0141	1.515	0.014793	0.0109	0.059194 (0.0172)	0.0408 (0.0811)
Malaysia	0.0067	1.541	-0.04367	-0.0121	0.042613 (0.070)	0.0416 (0.0760)
Mexico	0.0196	1.845	0.014193	-0.0134	0.060943 (0.0147)	0.0517 (0.0326)
Thailand	0.0083	2.122	0.004275	0.01126	0.048467 (0.0432)	0.0546 (0.0254)

6.4.2 Conditional valuation of assets with constant conditional betas

The test of the conditional version of the Sharpe-Lintner model is shown in table (5). This model assumes that expected asset returns are proportional to the expected return on the world market portfolio, efficient in the mean-variance sense. Beta is the weighting coefficient.

The highest betas were recorded in Hong Kong and Thailand. Austria and Argentina have the lowest betas. Standard deviations are fairly high for emerging markets, and betas are widely dispersed. The USA has a beta of 0.9781, while Japan has a beta of 0.8094. However, the differences in betas do not explain the differences in average excess returns, which are 0.72% for the USA and -0.02% for Japan.

With common variables, the model's hypotheses are rejected at the 5% level for Australia, Austria, Canada, the Netherlands and Indonesia. By introducing local variables, the model is rejected for the USA, the Netherlands, Chile and Thailand. In line with the general model, the null hypothesis is verified for the multivariate test, so the moment conditions are valid for both common and local information variables.

The table also shows the valuation errors based on estimates with common instrumental variables. The average error for the USA is -0.27%, implying that the model provides an average expected return of 0.99% per month and an average realized return of 0.72%. For Japan, the model predicts -0.41% returns, where only -0.02% is realized on average.

Table (5): Estimation of conditional CAPM with time varying expected returns and constant conditional betas

Emerging markets	β_j (standard deviation) (t-student)	Average yield	Average error	$\overline{R^2}$	Instruments common Hansen's J-statistic (*P-value*)	Local instruments Hansen's J-statistic (*P-value*)
Argentina	0.6412 (1.2915) (0.4965)	0.0231	-0.0202	0.0184	0.0193 (0.2802)	0.0188 (0.2690)
Chile	1.6158 (0.8257) (1.9567)	0.0125	-0.0051	0.0251	0.0362 (0.0615)	0.0426 (0.0343)
Korea	1.8092 (1.3166) (1.3741)	0.0083	-6.78E-05	0.0506	0.0364 (0.0601)	0.0271 (0.1376)
Indonesia	-1.2873 (2.0487) (-0.6283)	0.0141	-0.0200	0.0626	0.0401 (0.0429)	0.0284 (0.1228)
Malaysia	1.5242 (0.9178) (1.6606)	0.0067	0.0002	0.0191	0.0280 (0.1972)	0.0230 (0.1271)
Mexico	1.9092* (0.9901) (2.0100)	0.0196	-0.0105	0.0191	0.0357 (0.0644)	0.0356 (0.0649)
Thailand	2.3180 (1.4741) (1.5725)	0.0083	0.0022	0.0436	0.0359 (0.0627)	0.0525 (0.0136)

Developed Markets	β_j	Average yield	Average error	$\overline{R^2}$	Instruments common J-statistics	Local instruments J-statistics
Germany	1.2604* (0.4238) (2.9736)	0.0070	-0.0012	-0.0078	0.0118 (0.4928)	0.0134 (0.4352)
Australia	1.1812* (0.5086) (2.3221)	0.0059	-0.0005	0.0153	0.0424 (0.0347)	0.0321 (0.0882)

Austria	0.6123 (0.6217) (0.9848)	0.0074	-0.0046	0.0282	0.0386 (0.0494)	0.0187 (0.2841)
Belgium	1.1790* (0.4577) (2.5755)	0.0068	-0.0014	-0.0058	0.0210 (0.2343)	0.0283 (0.1246)
Canada	1.1331* (0.3805) (2.9779)	0.0060	-0.0008	0.0148	0.0401 (0.0429)	0.0205 (0.2434)
Spain	1.4089* (0.4957) (2.8418)	0.0060	-0.0003	-0.0135	0.0092 (0.5976)	0.0109 (0.5267)
United States	0.9781* (0.2265) (4.3174)	0.0072	-0.0027	0.0140	0.0353 (0.0662)	0.0431 (0.0327)
France	1.2841* (0.3409) (3.7657)	0.0068	-0.0020	0.0001	0.0206 (0.2420)	0.0291 (0.1158)
Hong Kong	2.1721* (0.8661) (2.5076)	0.0092	0.0007	-0.0120	0.0097 (0.5752)	0.0109 (0.5269)
Italy	0.9091 (0.5029) (1.8075)	0.0053	-0.0011	-0.0106	0.0124 (0.4719)	0.0252 (0.1621)
Japan	0.8094 (0.6540) (1.2375)	-0.0002	0.0039	0.0083	0.0321 (0.0883)	0.0323 (0.0867)
Netherlands	1.4054* (0.3401) (4.1313)	0.0065	-0.00013	0.0320	0.0419 (0.0365)	0.0410 (0.0396)
United Kingdom	0.7433* (0.2963) (2.5085)	0.0048	-0.0014	-0.0042	0.0222 (0.2110)	0.0224 (0.2070)
Sweden	1.8224* (0.5753) (3.1667)	0.0110	-0.0026	0.0047	0.0261 (0.3403)	0.0165 (0.1512)
Switzerland	1.4512* (0.4645) (3.1240)	0.0085	-0.0019	-0.0007	0.0268 (0.1419)	0.0233 (0.1915)
G7					0.1236 (0.2428)	0.1232 (0.2463)

6.4.3 Conditional asset valuation, case where the global price of covariance risk is constant

Table (6) shows the test of the model that assumes time-varying conditional covariances. The parameter λin the estimation represents the expected remuneration of world market volatility, i.e. the world price of covariance risk. However, in the estimates for individual countries, this parameter is not assumed to be constant. Using the common information variables, the model is rejected at the 5% level for Australia, Chile, Indonesia, Korea, Malaysia and Thailand, and at the 10% level for Mexico. With the exception of Korea and Hong Kong, the same result is obtained with local information variables.

The remuneration of the risk ratio varies considerably from country to country. The expected compensation for global market volatility is 5.0 in the USA and -1.40 in Japan. In a financially integrated global market, risk compensation should be the same in all countries. The last row of the table shows the test of the hypothesis that risk reward is constant between the different G7 countries. This measure, which is interpreted as the global price of risk covariance, is estimated at 3.34. It is almost equal to that of Italy and the UK, and lower than that of the other G7 countries (due to the presence of Japan). In the multivariate test, the hypothesis of the constancy of the world price of covariance risk is validated for both common and local information variables.

Table (6): Estimation of conditional CAPM with time-varying expected returns and constant price of covariance risk

Developed Markets	λ_j	Covariance average	Error average	Average yield	Error average	$\overline{R^2}$	Instruments common χ^2	Local instruments χ^2
Germany	4.4503 (2.5994)	0.0019	-0.0012	0.0070	0.0009	- 0.0120	0.0088 (0.6179)	0.0099 (0.5699)
Australia	2.1026 (2.3703)	0.0013	-0.0005	0.0059	-0.0033	0.0130	0.0653 (0.0041)	0.0676 (0.0032)
Austria	4.1986 (4.0145)	0.0010	-0.0046	0.0074	-0.0035	0.0150	0.0370 (0.0569)	0.0211 (0.2306)
Belgium	5.2796 (2.7343)	0.0013	-0.0014	0.0068	0.0005	- 0.0025	0.0266 (0.1438)	0.0284 (0.1235)
Canada	5.4620 (2.7106)	0.0015	-0.0008	0.0060	0.0023	0.0005	0.0350 (0.0680)	0.0320 (0.0892)
Spain	3.1205 (1.1248)	0.0019	-0.0003	0.0060	-0.0006	- 0.0107	0.0159 (0.3554)	0.0187 (0.2841)
United States	5.0015 (2.1939)	0.0014	-0.0027	0.0072	-0.0017	- 0.0101	0.0131 (0.4455)	0.0131 (0.4442)
France	4.7803 (2.3299)	0.001782	-0.0020	0.0068	-0.0002	- 0.0123	0.0119 (0.4903)	0.0126 (0.4628)
Hong Kong	5.2184 (3.0068)	0.0018	0.0007	0.0092	0.0005	0.0010	0.0336 (0.0771)	0.0402 (0.0427)
Italy	3.0738 (2.5934)	0.0016	-0.0011	0.0053	-0.0008	- 0.0095	0.0167 (0.3350)	0.0290 (0.1162)
Japan	-1.4022 (2.0779)	0.0019	0.0039	-0.0002	-0.0023	0.0048	0.0323 (0.0872)	0.0326 (0.0849)
Netherlands	4.4156 (2.0439)	0.0016	- 0.00013	0.0065	0.0006	0.0037	0.0275 (0.1337)	0.0295 (0.1113)
United Kingdom	3.0457 (1.5486)	0.0015	-0.0014	0.0048	-0.0001	- 0.0122	0.0125 (0.4675)	0.0132 (0.4425)
Sweden	6.6182 (2.6052)	0.0023	-0.0026	0.0110	0.0047	0.0008	0.0199 (0.2564)	0.0205 (0.2433)
Switzerland	6.4178 (2.6047)	0.0014	-0.0019	0.0085	0.0004	- 0.0038	0.0234 (0.1897)	0.0229 (0.1979)
G7	3.3425 (1.3338) (2.5059)						0.1319 (0.4751)	0.1221 (0.5860)

Emerging markets	λ_j	Covariance average	Error average	Average yield	Error average	$\overline{R^2}$	Instruments common χ^2	Local instruments χ^2
Argentina	-1.5832 (4.8206)	0.0001	-0.0202	0.0231	-0.0249	0.0073	0.0300 (0.1072)	0.0291 (0.1154)
Chile	16.3837 (5.4267)	0.0010	-0.0051	0.0125	0.0049	- 0.0130	0.0437 (0.0309)	0.0552 (0.0106)
Korea	3.0059 (3.4626)	0.0021	- 6.78E05	0.0083	-0.0009	0.0424	0.0444 (0.0290)	0.0356 (0.0645)
Indonesia	-2.7545 (5.6081)	0.0015	-0.0200	0.0141	-0.0183	0.0774	0.0566 (0.0092)	0.0417 (0.0372)
Malaysia	5.5102 (4.0379)	0.0015	0.0002	0.0067	0.0020	0.0121	0.0454 (0.0264)	0.0445 (0.0287)
Mexico	8.5629 (4.0655)	0.0018	-0.0105	0.0196	-0.0029	- 0.0119	0.0365 (0.0595)	0.0363 (0.0605)
Thailand	5.3547 (4.1205)	0.0021	0.0022	0.0083	0.0036	0.0244	0.0536 (0.0123)	0.0501 (0.0170)

SUMMARY

International financial integration is a central theme in international finance. Indeed, from the 1990s onwards, the degree of integration of emerging markets has increased significantly, due to the reduction in financials over the period 1987-2004. The results indicate that the global market portfolio is conditionally constrained by portfolio flows, capital market liberalization and the introduction of ADRs and country funds on US stock exchanges. In this work, three conditional versions of the International CAPM have been estimated using data for 22 efficient markets in the mean-variance sense for G7 countries, with the highest betas recorded in emerging financial markets. Estimation of the CAPM in the case where the global price of covariance risk is constant, indicates that risk remuneration varies considerably between the 22 countries examined. The global price of covariance risk is only constant for the G7 as a whole, so the financial integration hypothesis is only valid for the largest developed countries.

BIBLIOGRAPHICAL REFERENCES

Aglietta M., 1991, "L'ajustement international", Cahiers Français, October-December pp. 94-104.

Akdogan H., 1996, "A Suggested Approach to Country Selection in International Portfolio Diversification", Journal of Portfolio Management, 23, pp. 33-39.

Allen D., and G MacDonald, 1995, "The Long Run Gains from International Equity Diversification: Australian Evidence from Cointegration Tests", Applied Financial Economics, 5, pp. 33-42.

Aloui C., and N Bouanani, 2005, "Interdépendance et Co-mouvements des Marches des Capitaux des Pays Arabes de la Région du Moyen Orient et d'Afrique du Nord : Un Essai d'Investigation Empirique", Economic Research Forum, Working Paper 0316.

Amihud Y., and H Mendelson, 1986, "Asset Pricing and the Bid-Ask Spread" , Journal of Financial Economics, 17, pp. 223-247.

Ammer J., and J Mei, 1996, "Measuring International Economics Linkage with Stock Market Data", Journal of Finance, 51, pp. 1743-1763.

Anderson T G., 1996, "Return Volatility and Trading Volume", Journal of Finance, 51, pp.169-204.

Barari M., 2004, "Measuring Equity Market Integration Using Market Time-Varing Integration Score: The Case of Latin America", International Review of Financial Analysis, 13, pp.649-668.

Bekaert G., and Harvey C., 1995, "Time-Varying World Market Integration", Journal of Finance, 50, pp. 403-444.

Bekaert G., and Harvey C., 2000, "Foreign Speculator and Emerging Equity Markets", Journal of Finance, 55, pp. 565-615.

Bekaert G., and R Hodrick, 1992, "Characterizing Predictable Components in Excess Returns on Equity and Foreign Exchange Markets", Journal of Finance, 47, pp. 467-509.

Black F., 1972, "Capital Market Equilibrium with restricted borrowing", Journal of Business, 45, pp.444-455.

Campbel J Y., and R J Shiller, 1988, "The Dividend-price Ratio and Expectations of Future Dividends and Discount Factors", Review of Financial Studies, 1, pp. 195-228.

Campbel J Y., and Y Hamao. 1992, "Predictable Bond and Stock Returns in the United States and Japan: A Study of Long Term Capital Market Integration", Journal of Finance, 47, pp. 43-70.

Canova F., and G DeNicole, 1995, "Stock Returns and Real Activity: A Structural Approach", European Economic Review, 39, pp. 981-1015.

Carrieri F., V Errunza, and K Hogan, 2007, "Characterizing World Market Integration Through Time", Journal of Financial and Quantitative Analysis.

Chakravarty S., A Sarkar, and L F Wu, 1998. "Information Asymmetry, market Segmentation and Segmentation and Pricing of Cross-listed Shares: Theory and Evidence from Chinese A and B Shares," Working Paper, Purdue University.

Chen G.M., B.S Lcc, and O Rui, 2001, "Foreign Ownership Restrictions and Market Segmentation in China's Stock Markets", Journal of Financial Research, 14, pp. 133-155.

Cho D; C S Eun and L W Senbet, 1986, "International Arbitrage Pricing Theory: An Empirical Investigation", Journal of Finance, 41, pp. 313-330.

Davies A., 2006, "Testing for International Equity Market Integration Using Regime Switching Cointegration Techniques", Review of Financial studies, 15, pp. 305-321.

Dumas B., 1994, "A Test of International CAPM Using Business Cycles Indicators as Instrumental Variables", The Internationalization of Equity Markets, Jeffrey Frenkel Edition, University of Chicago, Press Chicago, pp. 23-50.

Dumas B., 1995, "Marché International des Capitaux : Modèles d'Equilibre Partiel contre Modèles d'Equilibre Général", Encyclopédie des Marchés Financiers, pp 803-845.

Dumas B., and B Solnik, 1995, "The World Price of Foreign Exchange Rate Risk". Journal of Finance, 50, pp. 445-479.

Engle R F., and C W J Granger, 1987, "Cointegration and Error Correction: Representation, Estimation and Testing" Econometrica, 55, pp. 251-276.

Errunza V., E Losq, and P Padmanabhan, 1992, "Tests of Integration, Mild Segmentation and Segmentation Hypotheses" , Journal of Banking and Finance, 16, pp. 949-972.

Errunza V., and D Miller., 2000, "Market Segmentation and Cost of Capital in International Equity Markets" Journal of Financial and Quantitative Analysis, 35, pp. 577-600.

Errunza V., and E Losq ., 1985, "International Asset Pricing under Mild Segmentation: Theory and Test", Journal of Finance, 40, pp. 105-124.

Errunza V., V Senbet, and K Hogan, 1998, "The Pricing of Country Funds from Emerging Markets: Theory and Evidence" International Journal of Theoretical and Applied Finance, 1, pp .111-143.

Eun C S., and S Janakiramanan, 1986, "A Model of International Asset Pricing with a Constraint on the Foreign Equity Ownership", Journal of Finance, 41, pp.897-914.

Eun C S., and S Shim, 1993, "International transmission of Stock Market Movements", International Financial Market Integration, S R Stansell Edition, Blackwell, pp.259-277.

Fama EF., and K R French., 1988, "Dividend Yields and Expected Stock Returns", Journal of Financial Economics, 22, pp. 3-25.

Ferson W E . and C R Harvey, 1994, "Sources of Risk and Expected Returns in Global Equity Markets", Journal of Banking and Finance, 18, pp.775-803.

Ferson W E .,and C R Harvey. 1991, "The Variation of Economic Risk Premiums", Journal of

Foerester S R., and G A Karolyi, 1999, "The effects of Market Segmentation and Investor Recognition on Asset Prices: Evidence from Foreign Stocks Listing in the United States", Journal of Finance, 4, pp. 981-1013.

Fontaine P., 1988, "Arbitrage et Evaluation Internationale des actifs financiers", Edition Economica, Paris.

Frankel J., 1991, "Quantifying International Capital Mobility in the 1980s", In D. Bernheim and J. Shoven, eds. National Savings and Economic Performance, pp. 227-260.

Frankel J., and A T MacArthur, 1988, "Political vs. Currency Premia in International Real Interest Rate Differentials: A study of Forward Rates of 24 Countries", European Economic Review, 32, pp 1083-1121.

Fratzcher M., 2002, "Financial Market Integration in Europe: on the Effects of EMU on Stock Markets", International Journal of Finance and Economics, 7, pp. 165-193.

Grauer F L A., R H Litzenberger, and R S Stehle, 1976, "Sharing Rules and Equilibrium in an International Capital Market under Uncertainty", Journal of Financial Economics, 3, pp. 233-256.

Gultekin M N., and N B Gultekin, 1983, "Stock Market Seasonality: International Evidence", Journal of Financial Economics, 12, pp. 469-481.

Gultekin M N., N B Gultekin, and A Penati, 1989, "Capital Controls and International Capital Market Segmentation: the Evidence from the Japanese and American Stock Markets", Journal of Finance, 44, pp. 849-869.

Hamao Y., 1988, "An Empirical Examination of the Arbitrage Pricing Theory: Using Japanese Data", Japan and the World Economy, 1, pp. 45-61.

Hamilton J D., 1990, "Analysis of Time Series Subject to Changes in Regime Application to the ISLM Model", Journal of Econometrics, 45, pp. 39-70.

Hansen L P., 1982, "Large Sample properties of Generalized Method of Moments Estimators", Econometrica, 50, pp. 1029-1054.

Hardouvelis G D., S Straetmans, and C De Vries, 1999, "EMU and European Stock Market Integration", CEPR Discussion Paper, no. 2124.

Harvey C R ., B Solnik, and G Zhou, 1994, "What Determines Expected International Asset Returns? Working paper , Duke University, Durham.

Harvey C R., 1991, "The World Price of Covariance Risk", Journal of Finance, 4pp. 111-157.

Henry P., 1998, "Do Stock Market Liberalizations Cause Investment Booms: Evidence from the Finnish Market", Journal of Financial Economics, 16, pp. 33-53.

Hietala P T., 1989, "Asset Pricing in Partially Segmented Markets: Evidence from the Finnish Market", Journal of Financial Economics, 36, pp. 3-27.

Hunter D M., 2007, "The Evolution of Stock Market Integration in the Post-Liberalization Period: A Look of Latin America", Journal of International Money and Finance, 25, pp. 795-826.

Jagannathan R., and Z Wang, 1996, "The Conditional CAPM and the Cross-Section of Expected Returns", Journal of Finance, 51, pp. 3-53.

Jong F., and F A De Roon, 2005, "Time Varying Market Integration and Expected Returns in Emerging Markets", Journal of Financial Economics, 78, pp. 583-613.

Jorion P., and E Schwartz, 1986, "Integration Versus Segmentation in the Canadian Stock Market", Journal of Finance, 41, pp. 603-617.

Keim D B., 1983, "Size Related Anomalies and Stock Return Seasonality", Journal of Financial Economics, 12, pp. 13-32.

Kim S J., F Moshirian, and E Wu, 2006, "Evolution of International Stock and Bond Market Integration: Influence of the European Monetary Union", Journal of Banking and Finance, 30, pp 1507-1534.

King M., and S Wadhani, 1990, "Transmission of Volatility Between Stock Markets", Review of Financial Studies, 3, pp. 5-33.

Korajczyk R., and C Viallet, 1989, "An Empirical Investigation of International Asset Pricing", Review of Financial Studies, 2, pp. 553-585.

Koutmos G., and G Booth, 1995, "AsymmetricVolatility Transmission in International Stock Markets", Journal of International Money and Finance, 14, pp. 747-762.

La Bruslerie H De., and J Mathis, 1997, "Intégration Partielle des Marchés Financiers Internationaux : Modélisation et Test Empirique", Annales d'Economie et de Statistique, 46, pp.115-139.

Lintner J., 1965, "The Valuation of Risk Assets and the Selection of Risky Investment in Stock Portfolios and Capital Budgets", Review of Economics and Statistics, 47, pp. 103-124.

Ng A., 2000, "Volatility Spillover Effects from Japan and the US to the Pacific-Basin", Journal of International Money and Finance, 19, pp. 207-233.

Phylaktis K., and F Ravazzolo, 2002, Measuring Financial and Economic Integration with Equity Prices in Emerging Markets, Journal of International Money and Finance, 21, pp. 879-904.

Piesse J., and Hearn B., 2002, "Equity Market Integration versus Segmentation in Three Dominant Markets of the Southern African Customs Union: Cointegration and Causality Tests", Applied Economics, 34, pp. 1711-1722.

Roll R., 1992, "Industrial Structure and the Comparative Behavior of International Stock Market Indices", Journal of Finance, 47, pp. 3-41.

Schwert GW., 1990, "Stock Returns and Real Activity: A century of Evidence", Journal of Finance, 45, pp.1237-1257.

Sharpe W., 1964, "Capital Asset Prices: A Theory of Market Equilibrium under Conditions of Risk", Journal of Finance, 19, pp.425-442.

Solnik B., 1974, "An Equilibrium Model of the International Capital Market", Journal of Economic Theory, 8, pp. 111-157.

Solnik B., 1983, "International Arbitrage Pricing Theory", Journal of Finance, 38, pp. 449-457.

Stehle R., 1977, "An Empirical Test of the Alternative Hypothesis of National and International Pricing of Risky Assets", Journal of Finance, 32, pp. 493-503.

Stulz R., 1981a, "A Model of International Asset Pricing Model", Journal of Financial Economics, 9, pp. 383-406.

Stulz R., 1981b, "On the Effects of Barriers to International Investment", Journal of Finance, 36, pp. 923-934.

Stulz R., 1999, "Globalisation of Equity Markets and the Cost of Capital", Working Paper, Ohio State University.

Stulz R., and Wasserfallen W., 1995, "Foreign Equity Investment, Restrictions, Capital Flight and Shareholder Wealth Maximisation: Theory and Evidence", Review of Financial Studies, 8, pp. 1019-1057.

Tai C S., 2007, "Market Integration and Currency Risk in Asian Emerging Market", Research in International Business and Finance, 21, pp. 98-117.

Wheatley S., 1988, "Some Tests of International Equity Integration", Journal of Financial Economics, 21, pp. 177-212.

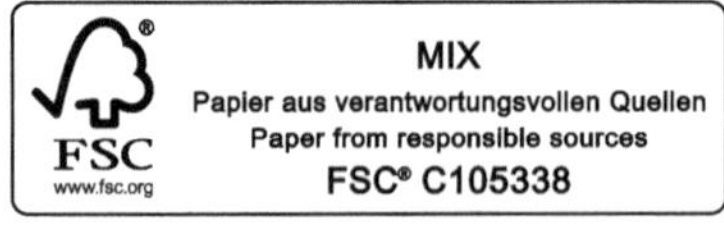

Printed by Books on Demand GmbH, Norderstedt / Germany